ROOKIE DAD

What to Expect During Your Partner's Pregnancy

CONTENTS

INTRODUCTION

When my wife became pregnant with our first child, I was the happiest I'd ever been. That pregnancy, labor, and birth were a period of amazing intimacy, sensitivity, and passion. Long before we married, my wife and I agreed to share equally in parenting our children. And it seemed only logical that the process of shared parenting begins during pregnancy.

However, even though this was our first child together, my wife already had four children from a prior marriage , who were now fifteen, seventeen, twenty-three, and twenty-five years old. So, my wife had experience with having children, but I had ZERO. This was my very first pregnancy. I was truly a "Rookie Dad." I realized that I didn't have a clue about pregnancies, babies, or kids, and the only thing I knew to do was to start reading as much information on the subject as possible.

I started looking for answers in my wife's pregnancy books, but the information regarding what expecting dads go through was, shall we say, cursory and consisted largely of advice on how men may be supportive of their pregnant spouses. As I read through several pregnancy books, and online resources, I started noticing that most of the information I read was written for the pregnant woman. It was obvious to me that us new dads were being left out.

Until recently, there has been very little study on pregnant dads' emotional and psychological experiences during pregnancy.

With that stated, and as you will soon discover, an expecting father's experience throughout the transition to fatherhood is not limited to general enthusiasm. If it were, this book would never have been written. The truth is that men's emotional reactions to pregnancy can vary far more than women. Expectant dads experience a range of emotions, from relief and joy to denial, dread, some amount of annoyance, and wrath—so you best brace yourself for what's to come, champ. I'd also want to mention that up to eighty percent of males experience physical pregnancy symptoms.

With those facts stated, it begs the question why in the world have we males been denied information? In my opinion, this is because we as a society value motherhood more than fatherhood, and we instinctively believe that women's childbirth and childbearing difficulties are the same. But, as you will discover, both by reading this book and by personal experience, this is simply not the case.

WHAT IS THE STRUCTURE OF THIS BOOK?

Throughout the book, I aim to give plain, practical information in an easy-to-digest fashion. Each of the key chapters is broken into sections–this was done since I am writing the book NOW, and my ideas flowed with enthusiasm during the time I was writing this book.

WHAT'S HAPPENING TO YOUR PARTNER?

Despite the fact that this book is about us dads. You still need to know what's going on with your spouse; check in with her to see how she's dealing with her pregnancy and how you can help. It is critical that you are aware of what your spouse is going through and when. As a result, I believe it is critical that we begin with what a woman truly encounters when she is carrying that kid in her stomach–so that you get a full understanding of what is going on.

THE BABY?

This section updates you on the growth of your future child, from sperm to egg to a live, breathing newborn, which is a moment that brings us men delight and a breath of fresh air.

Chapter

1

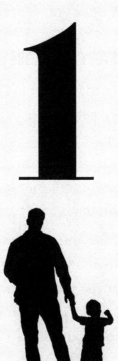

GROWING UP: MY CHILDHOOD, THE 80S KID, AND MY HOMETOWN; FRUITVILLE.

Expectation:

Among the first big decisions you and your spouse will face after learning she's pregnant are: How do we want to raise this child? Where are we going to have the baby? Who will help us deliver it? Will our money last? To some extent, the answers will be defined by the limits of your insurance coverage, but there are still a range of options to consider. As you consider your alternatives, give your spouse at least fifty-one percent of the vote. After all, the final decision affects her more than it does you.

A LITTLE STORY ABOUT THIS SURE DAD

I grew up in Fruitville, Florida, Sarasota county's suburbs. When I was a kid, I was a very active and inquisitive child. My pals would bother our neighbor, who had enormous plantations of orange trees. Yes, we loved and admired oranges, but when you grow up in an environment that has a plentiful crop of it all year, you feel it's something to play with.

However, my buddies and I would frequently trespass into a large orange grove and play baseball with the falling oranges, shattering them as soon as they hit our baseball bats. Matt and Ray were two of my closest friends. Their comments while we played that ingenious game in old Mr. Sam's yard still ring in my brain.

"Hey, pass the ball, you jerk," Matt would yell, and I'd toss it with my best shot. Not at the glove but at his face. The 'ball' would splatter and spread its juices all over Matt's face the moment it struck him.

Ray and I would laugh so hard that our ribs hurt. Matt would insist that we play again, not for the sake of entertainment but so that he could exact his childish vengeance. He would triumph, though, since we tolerated fair play in our group.

Mr. Sam owned the orange orchard; he was an older guy in his sixties at the time. We dubbed him "the creep master" because he would sneak up on us while we were playing so he could swat our buttocks. But we were wiser than him, the moment we noticed him nearby, we knew one of us had to keep an eye on him, so he didn't surprise us with the slipper he carried while following us. So, as soon as we noticed him, we left–*poof*. We would run so much that our rear legs could be felt. Mr. Sam would always exclaim that if he caught us, we would be sorry.

However, once we'd had our fun for the day, we had to be back home for dinner–before nightfall–this was a directive from our fathers, and mine was particularly severe about it.

However, I have fond recollections of my father. He was a superb disciplinarian, but he was also a workaholic. My favorite memory is playing baseball with him, where I played the catcher, and he always handled the baseball bat. We'd play for about thirty minutes on Saturday because the other days he was mostly busy on something and rarely came to play. We spent the rest of the weekend either playing baseball (as I mentioned) or watching football and baseball.

My mom would parade about with the laundry bag, and one day while my dad and I were watching a football game, he got up and walked over to my mother. I figured they were simply having an adult conversation, and I couldn't care less. I sat munching on popcorn and my favorite pepperoni pizza–mmm, that gooey sweetness. I still believe that pizzas from the 1970s and 1980s were far superior to those available now.

He didn't come back for me as I waited for him so we could continue watching the football game. When I initially grew anxious and began looking for him, I found him in the kitchen, chopping carrots. I didn't think such behavior was unusual, it was what a father did. But I found that wasn't the case when talking with friends when I was in my teens. They would constantly remind me how women had to stay at home to take care of their family while the father had to go to work and provide the finances for the family.

As a youngster, that didn't make sense to me. My father was always 'all hands-on deck' while he was at home with my mom and me. He'd tend to anything that would cause my mother concern. I'd implore my dad to simply sit and let Mom do the job, but he'd refuse and even force me to do the chores with him.

I always assumed it was some type of punishment and felt awful that my mother made us do the labor. Because after she was finished with hers, my dad and I would still be doing our tasks while she watched one of her favorite fashion programs.

But as I grew older, I realized that what my father was doing was the correct way to be a man and raise a family. My parents seldom disagreed, though there was the occasional little dispute. They found a method to manage family and personal difficulties. Some of my acquaintances had divorced fathers and mothers, but mine remained together till the end.

Then, as I grew older, I realized that my father's ways were exactly as things should be. Partners must support each other in order for the family to flourish in all areas, as well as for the man in the family to grow personally.

One day, my mother and I were viewing a videotape of me as a toddler, and in the film, I could see my father picking me up and playing with me while my mother reclined with her juice in hand—she was on a picnic mat, all fresh and youthful, with no worries in the world, while my father took part in playing with me.

Then the scene changed, and I saw my father changing my diapers. My mother chuckled and showed him how to do it, and all I could see was this synergy. They were content with their work. There was no guilt, only complete bliss.

By the time I graduated from high school, I wanted to be like my father. Because of that one act of his, I treated women as equals, giving them the respect, they deserved. You can imagine the mental balance that had on me as I grew up to the age of becoming a man and seeking for a partner myself.

However, when I married my wife and she became pregnant a year later, I was terrified since I had no idea what to anticipate. But I stuck to my father's ideas and traditions, assuring myself that no matter what happened at home, I would take care of my wife and treat her with complete respect, providing her with all the assistance she required.

My father was the best parent someone could possibly have. The way he governed his family with love and compassion was great for all of us.

Everyone in that house had a task. They had to work and assist mom, and that one attitude and law that my father passed on made my mom deliciously fresh and cheerful every single day of her life.

My elder sister—I failed to mention that I am the youngest of two older sisters—once told me about a time when I filled my diaper as a youngster. Mom was busy, and my younger sister didn't want to change my diaper. My mother was on the verge of a mental breakdown, having to cook, wash, and do a variety of other tasks while my father was abroad. I, on the other hand, was sobbing uncontrollably, especially because of my soiled diaper.

Fortunately, my father returned home just in time, when he noticed my mother on the sofa, clutching her face as if weeping. When he heard me crying, he raced over to me and began working without any instruction. My sisters observed how he was gentle with me. As soon as he removed the diaper, he directed Holly, my oldest sister, to hand him a clean one. Holly retrieved a clean diaper and handed it to him, and without hesitation he got to work. He washed my butt, adjusted the diaper, positioned it, and clipped it. It was quick!

As soon as he was finished, I burst out laughing, as happy as a newborn that I could finally feel at ease. Holly and Tracy often tell me that one deed from our father left an impression on them. They grew up to be responsible in order to meet responsible men who would be like my father and support them. And they weren't the only ones observed my father act like a 'super dad.' His actions left an indelible imprint on my memory that I will never forget.

As I grew older, my father and I grew closer. We'd have the nicest father-son times, especially on weekends.

Lesson Here:

- A father is expected to be humble and to treat his family with care and consideration.

Chapter

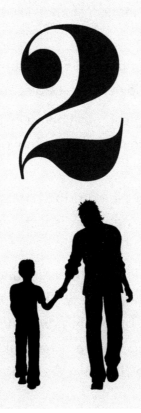

KING OF THE CASTLE, TOUGH LOVE:
THE DYNAMIC BETWEEN MY FATHER AND I

A decent father is unquestionably a child's most ardent supporter. It is quite wonderful when a caring parent makes his children feel as though he enjoys being around them. Every child may benefit from an excellent mother, but there is something especially unique between fathers and their sons.

Don't get me wrong: this isn't to mean that a person who doesn't have a strong connection with their father can't feel loved and satisfied via other forms of relationships—far from it. But when you have a fantastic father, like I had, you don't want to take it for granted.

A good father can make his son feel not just adored and humorous, but also powerful, capable, and smart.

This was true for me. I recall being in junior high; I had just graduated from grade school and was worried about entering a new period of my life.

As I walked down the corridor, I noticed students my age and older gazing at me with disgust. I was nervous, forged ahead.

While walking to class, three taller and older guys passed me and began laughing loudly. They laughed so loudly that it threw me off, and I thought it was incredibly impolite. To prevent them picking on me, I had taken a turn around a corner, but they yanked my hair and dragged me down to the floor.

Everyone in the corridor started laughing. Being picked on on my first day of school was not enjoyable and struck my confidence down. I jumped up, brushed off my shirt, and scrambled away from the bullies. Then went right to the bathroom, bawling my eyes out.

So, after class that day, my dad picked me up, as he always did. I got inside the car and remained silent for quite some time. My father suspected something was wrong, but I didn't want to tell him what had happened at school because I didn't want to appear weak. My father had always thought of me as a strong, self-assured young man. And, at the time, I believed I had learnt a lot from him to apply to the world, but I was completely mistaken. The world was far stronger than my feeble feelings, and I was no match for it.

"What's wrong?" he asked as he swung the car around a corner.

I remained mute since I didn't want to say anything. "Nothing, sir," I slouched.

"It is evident that something is amiss with my excellent man," he stated. "Didn't you enjoy school?"

I attempted to smile as I glanced up at him. I tried all I could to fake a grin, but I couldn't pull it off. I nodded, not knowing how to react. "I enjoyed school."

He grinned. "You don't have to lie to me, you know." He added, "You can tell me what's wrong, and I'll tell you what to do."

I started crying the instant he said it. It was really painful since I was lying to my father. My father was kind; he simply patted me on the back to let it all out.

Then he went to a shopping center, parked his car, and urged me to talk. He asked me to tell him everything that had happened so that he could figure out how he could assist.

"Some big boys were picking on me at school, dad," I explained. "I don't think anyone likes me at that school, since when the boys did it, none stopped them. They just laughed at me like I was a joke." Then I wiped my eyes and exhaled in satisfaction that I had told him and let it all out.

"Is that all?" he asked quietly.

"Yes, Dad," I said. "I'm sorry I lied to you at first; I didn't want you to feel like all of the teachings you taught me at home were for naught."

He then laughed. I recall my father chuckling every time we talked, as we still do.

"Good son, you're welcome to be human," he remarked after a few minutes of laughter.

I didn't get it. Welcome to be human? What did he mean? "Dad, what do you mean?" I inquired.

"That's life," he responded. "We all have our experiences, some good, some bad. But you have to determine how you want to react to the uncool or difficult stuff."

I didn't get it. How should you respond to the uncool stuff? If I had the chance, I would have removed all of the uncool stuff and left only the cool. "Dad, I just want the cool stuff; how can I have it?" I enquired.

"Your attitude, my little kid," he responded. "All you have to show them is that you're the boss and their laughing doesn't frighten you."

I was attentive. "So, I can select not to be a joke to anyone?"

He nodded. "Life is made up of the attitudes we give it," he remarked. "If you agree you're a joke to everybody, including your colleagues at school, then they'll take you as a joke during your tenure at that school. But if you show them that you're in charge, you'll get their respect, as well as some wonderful friends who may wish to rely on you."

I longed for friends as a kid. So, when he mentioned it to me, it piqued my interest. So, with my dad's guidance, I might be able to form my own group at school! That comment stuck in my head, and I made the firm decision to carry out this strategy the following day at school.

"Are you cool now?" he questioned.

I smiled as I nodded. I was a featherweight and reverted to my previous self. I couldn't wait for tomorrow to show all those students what I had.

"All right, then, let me get you some ice cream," he replied, and we both hopped out of the car, giddy.

Fortunately for me, I have an excellent father. My father made certain that I was never made to feel bad about my unpleasant ideas, feelings, and opinions. He congratulated me whenever he spotted me doing anything nice or working hard. When I told him stories, he listened intently. When I was present, he said nice things about me to other grownups.

The next day, I went to school and implemented my father's instruction. I walked into school as if I owned it. Most of the youngsters were perplexed by my stride or how I could walk so tall and mighty despite yesterday's shame.

My father was my supporter. He was always the man I looked to for counsel. Even now, I approach him to seek guidance on how to efficiently manage my house. When I needed it, my father corrected me as well. I was never a spoiled brat—never. He wanted me to act in a way that was consistent with my good character. As encouraging as he was, he kept me grounded. He managed to make me feel great without making me believe I was above the rules or better than anybody else.

He encouraged me with a purpose. My father never once told me that things I tried wasn't my gift but carefully and tenderly steered me to areas he felt I was more suited.

Here's one I recall distinctly. Scott Danish, a buddy of mine, once taught me how to draw cartoons. I like sketching but wasn't particularly good at it. But I aspired to be like my friend Scott. As a child, I was impressed by the ease with which he drew those lines. He could sketch anything, and I mean anything, even our favorite action figures, with ease. I told Scott to teach me, but no matter how hard I tried to draw those lines and figures as he did, I never truly measured up to his talent, which irritated me.

So, one day I arrived home irritated and feeling worthless. Mom was busy with my sister's hair as I sat on the living room floor thinking about how worthless I was. Fortunately for me, dad returned home that day—before that dreadful notion could sink in any deeper. He sat for a time, observing me while I struggled with the pen and paper.

"What are you doing, kiddo?" he said, tossing his luggage on the sofa and sitting to watch me fight with that wretched pen.

"I want to sketch," I explained. "But I don't know how, and a guy at my school draws far better than I do."

He became silent for a while when he watched me draw the line, and I flopped, tore the paper, dumped it in the trash, and started over.

"But is this truly necessary?" he wondered.

I gave him a short nod with that kid-like grumbling, and he grinned. "I don't have any skills, and it makes me unhappy," I grumbled.

"Oh, no," he said. "Who says you don't have many talents?"

"Me," I said naively. "I want to draw like Scott, but no matter how hard I try, I fail."

"That's because you don't need to be him," my father explained. "Have you thought of coloring?"

"I can color rather well," I said.

"Does Scott know how to color?" he inquired.

"I don't think so, but he draws so beautifully," I responded.

"Then there's something you do that Scott doesn't know how to do," he quickly informed me, and it dawned on me that he was telling the truth—so, really, I did have skill, and it encouraged me.

"Thank you, Dad," I said. "That feels better." And I gave him a big embrace in thanks and to welcome him back.

I want to thank him here for protecting me from all the problems that come with being a kid. Thank you, Dad, for always being there when I needed you the most.

My father proudly displayed my assignments at his desk when I began to show potential as a writer. He was extremely proud of me, and his pride gave me the courage to think I was as intelligent as he claimed. I excelled in every enjoyable and informative activity at school, and I never fell behind.

But no matter how close we have always been, I have never been "Daddy's little boy." I was never a spoiled or pampered brat. If I did something wrong, he would correct me right away. I was always simply his son. He treated me as though I was intelligent, talented, and powerful.

My father never conveyed any grief to me as I grew older. Maybe he felt melancholy as I transitioned from a tiny boy to a young man, but I never knew. He simply remained by my side the entire time, assisting me in figuring out how to deal with whatever occurred next. My father guided me through all of the bullying, betrayals, and grief of my adolescence.

Our connection evolved naturally as I grew older. He began speaking to me as if I were an adult with the ability to make my own decisions. I'm sure he felt all the mixed feelings that come with watching your child leave the nest, but he always made me feel free to do my own thing.

I'm forty years old now, and I still chat to my "pops guy" every day. I've realized that my friendship with him has taught me some of the most crucial lessons in life. And here are a few of them that may be of use to you:

1. We don't always get it right:

My father worked many jobs while still supporting my mother at home. In reality, my father worked two jobs: one in the office and one at home. And he did it cheerfully and gladly; he was never forced to do anything.

His personal route, on the other hand, has shifted dramatically throughout the course of his life. He didn't care what path I took as long as I was doing something important that made me happy.

He paid for my private school education my whole childhood, yet he rarely stressed the need of college. He was encouraging when I decided to go to college. He was also cool with me dropping out before I finished my degree. Any life I chose was fine with my father, as long as I was happy and able to support my family. I've also taken some stupid chances that turned out perfectly because I knew he'd try his best to help me refocus if it didn't work out.

2. I am worthy to be respected and I shouldn't settle for less:

My connection with my father established the standard for how I should be treated by others. I'm convinced that having a close relationship with my father helped me choose a decent partner. I've never had to demand respect from my wife. She is the type of person who treats others decently.

Because of my father, I feel I quickly identified my wife as a wonderful choice for a life mate. When I first saw her, I noticed an atmosphere of respect around her that reminded me of my parents, especially my father. Everything about her made me think about somebody in my family, and I decided right then and there to make her my life partner. And I've never regretted it since. My wife and father have a common trait: they support each other in the family and believe in mutual respect.

3. *I decide the path of my Life:*

When I was married, I waited at the altar while my father stood a few feet away, in the first chair, cheering me on. That's my father; he trusted me to make the best decisions. I also knew that if I changed my mind, his keys would be in his pocket, and he was ready to drive me home. He wanted anything I wanted for myself.

His faith in me has led me to believe in myself. I am aware that I am the sole authority on myself. I know who I am and who I am not. Of course, I confer with others, when necessary, but I ultimately trust myself to know what is best for me.

It would be unjust to pretend that our lovely relationship has been flawless. That would undermine the deliberate method in which we choose to forgive one another for our imperfections in order to remain a team.

Yes, my father is not a perfect man, and I am not the ideal son. We have maintained a strong friendship to this day, but it has not been without flaws. We've evolved through some opposing viewpoints over time, and there are certain issues on which we just don't agree. We've also both made decisions that have disappointed the other.

Regardless, we always find a way to agree and put our differences to rest. I am a thankful man, and I am glad that the Lord gave me to such a man!

Lesson:

- A decent father is unquestionably a child's most ardent supporter.

- A good father can make his son feel not just adored and humorous but also powerful, capable, and smart.

Have faith in your child and trust that he or she will always do the right thing. As a result, you will be known as the "best father."

Chapter

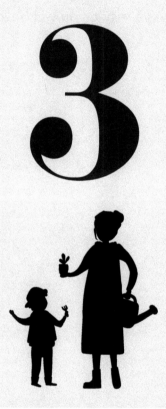

3

MOTHER PREPPER, THE EXPERIENCED MOTHER

The Where and the How State of Things

My wife was no newcomer to this. She'd had four children before my son was born.

Most couples, especially first-time parents, give birth in a hospital. It is also, in many people's opinion, the safest. In the uncommon event that difficulties emerge, most hospitals have experts on call twenty-four hours a day and are fully stocked with life-saving equipment and pharmaceuticals.

And, during the initial frenetic hours or days after the delivery, the on-staff nurses monitor the baby and mother and assist both new parents with the thousands of questions that are bound to arise. They also like creating havoc for you and fending off undesirable intruders. If you have a choice of hospitals in your region, I recommend that you go on a tour of each one before making your pick.

Most of the time, you will wind up going to the hospital where your partner's doctor or midwife has privileges—or the hospital where your insurance plan directs you to go. Some individuals choose the hospital first, then look for a practitioner who is affiliated with that facility.

Many hospitals now offer their own birth rooms, or even birthing facilities, where the patient's sole purpose is to bring someone into the world. These birth rooms are meticulously arranged to appear less antiseptic and medical and more like a bedroom at home, giving the overall impression of a lovely hotel suite or a cute bed and breakfast. The warm decor is intended to put you and your companion at rest. But the wood furniture skillfully hiding unique monitoring systems, the cabinet full of clean supplies, and the nurses dropping in every hour or so to give your spouse a pelvic exam will make it difficult to forget where you are. Keep in mind that some hospitals assign delivery rooms on a first come-first-serve basis, so don't bank on receiving one unless you can convince your spouse to go into labor before anybody else does that day. In other hospitals, all labor rooms are also birth rooms, and thus this would not be an issue.

Most hospitals are, by definition, bustling institutions with a slew of regulations and policies that may or may not make sense to you. Giving birth in a hospital usually means less privacy for you and your partner and more regular procedures for her and the baby.

With that said, if your partner is considered "high risk," which may mean she's carrying twins or more, is over thirty, has had complications in the past, especially during delivery, has medical risk factors, or was told anything that might be of concern by her practitioner, then a hospital birth should be the only option here.

ISOLATED BIRTHING CENTERS

Of the one to two percent of deliveries that occur outside of a hospital, over thirty percent occur in private or secluded birth facilities. These are staffed by certified nurse-midwives (CNMs), and they provide a more personalized approach to the delivery process. They have a homey atmosphere to them, with excellent decor, a kitchen, and hot tubs. They are often more flexible than hospitals and more willing to meet any requirements your spouse may have.

For example, there are less routine medical exams of any kind, your partner may be permitted to eat during labor—something that many hospitals prohibit—and she may be able to wear the clothing she prefers. There is no reason for her to wear those ugly dresses unless she truly desires one.

The personnel, on the other hand, will make every effort to ensure that your partner and infant are never separated. One disadvantage is that you and your newly extended family may need to check out as soon as six to ten hours following birth.

Private birth clinics are designed to handle simple, low-risk pregnancies and deliveries, so expect to be prescreened. And don't worry: if anything doesn't go as planned, birth facilities are always linked with a doctor and are frequently affiliated to a hospital or only a short ambulance ride away.

If you are interested in investigating this option, all you need to do is obtain the proper reference from your spouse's practitioner or friends and relatives.

HOME BIRTH

With all of their high-tech efficiency and austere, impersonal, sterile environments, hospitals aren't for everyone. As a result, some couples—roughly fewer than one percent—decided to deliver their baby at home. Home birth has been practiced for a long time (before 1920 was the period of most home births). However, it has been out of favor in America for a long time. It is, however, making a return, with most of my friends having already or are going to follow this path of birth.

My wife and I considered having our son at home, but we eventually opted against it. While I'm not especially squeamish, I couldn't understand how we'd avoid creating a mess all over the bedroom carpet and my favorite living space. What sealed the deal for us was that my wife was in her 40s and considered a "high risk" pregnancy. So, we chose the hospital setting to be safe.

Now, if you're considering a home birth, you'll need to be prepared—and I mean extremely prepared. Having a baby at home is not at all what it was in the ancient days, or in the old western times when ladies would be on the farm and pull the baby out of their pelvis. You will need to take far more responsibility for the entire procedure than if you used a hospital. It requires a lot of study and planning. You'll need a lot more than just clean towels and hot water.

Making the decision to give birth at home does not mean that your spouse may forgo prenatal care or that the two of you can plan on delivering your baby alone. You will still need to keep in constant touch with a medical expert to ensure that the pregnancy is proceeding correctly, and you should have someone there for the delivery who has had a lot of experience with birthing. And please, I don't mean your sister or mother-in-law, unless they are trained and certified. If not, it would be dangerous for your spouse. So, if you decide to go this route, start looking for a midwife right away.

Though statistically unlikely, if you are thinking about it, I want to walk you through some of the most frequent reasons people choose to have their child at home and some of the things that would make such births dangerous.

People choose to give birth at home for a variety of reasons:

- It is far less expensive, and the surroundings are more familiar, pleasant, and private.

- Hospitals are notorious for being overrun with sick

people.

- You've previously had one or more simple hospital deliveries.
- You can surround yourself with anybody you choose.
- You may focus on the spiritual elements of childbirth, something you may be discouraged from or feel ashamed about at the hospital.
- You dislike physicians and hospitals, or you are terrified of them.
- The circumstances are more familiar, comfortable, and private.
- If you had a horrible experience with a prior childbirth.

Reasons not to have a baby at home:

- No insurance coverage.
- She has a medical problem, such as diabetes or a renal ailment, or she has had a hemorrhage during childbirth, or she smokes, or she has had a previous cesarean section.
- Your partner is over the age of thirty-five or has been warned by her doctor that she is a "high risk."
- She goes into labor early.
- She's pregnant with twins or more. Or you discover that the baby is breech, that is; feet down instead of head down.
- She developed preeclampsia, a disease that affects around ten percent of pregnant women and can lead

to catastrophic complications if not recognized and treated early enough.

Now that we are through with that, let's talk of **Natural versus Medicated Birth**

Giving birth "naturally" without drugs, pain, medicine, or any other medical intervention has become vogue in recent years. However, just because something is popular does not mean it is appropriate for everyone. Labor and delivery will be a terrible experience for both of you, though in different ways, and many couples choose to take advantage of medical improvements in alleviating pain and suffering associated with childbirth.

Regardless, make sure the choice is made by your spouse. Supporters of some birthing approaches are almost obsessively dedicated to the notion of a drug-free delivery, to the point where they frequently make women who choose any pain medicine feel like failures. Aside from making many new parents feel horrible about themselves when they should be enjoying the birth of their child, such a hardline attitude is just out of touch with reality. Nationally, roughly half of women give birth with an epidural, which is the most popular form of pain treatment, and in certain large-city hospitals the percentage is as high as eighty-five percent.

There are benefits and drawbacks to both medicated and unmedicated deliveries, which we will discuss as we approach the baby's due date. But, for the time being, the most essential thing is to remain flexible and not let your friends, relatives, or anybody else put you under pressure to do anything you don't want to do.

Yes, you and your spouse may be anticipating a natural delivery, but problems may arise that demand intervention or the use of drugs. On the other hand, you may be planning a medicated birth but find yourself snowed in somewhere far from your hospital and any pain medicine, or the anesthesiologist may be at an emergency on the opposite side of town.

MY PERSONAL EXPERIENCE

When my wife and I were preparing for our son's birth, we considered our insurance coverage, the type of hospital that would be appropriate for our case, and a variety of other factors. I wanted to lead the way on handling those areas, so she would be as stress-free as possible, but I knew I didn't have any experience with it. She would know what to discuss, and what questions to ask.

My wife was a week late when we went for a visit, thinking the doctor would finally find a softer cervix and some dilation, but there was none. The baby was just where he wanted to be.

In times like these, you have to put on a good front because you don't want to leave your spouse with the impression that anything is going to go wrong. So, always keep a cheerful demeanor, and don't be too hard on yourself if you feel you don't have a solution to one or two issues when it comes to childbirth. However, luckily for you, I'm going to spell out all my experiences here and the steps I took, such as the things that need to be done and the food that needs to be eaten to make that baby healthy.

Who is Going to Help in the Process?

At first look, it appeared that my partner should choose a medical practitioner on her own—after all, she was the one who would be examined and prodded as the pregnancy approached its end. But, as I was informed by some nurses when I came in for checkups at various intervals, about 90 percent of today's expectant fathers are present during the delivery of their children, and the vast majority of them have been involved in a major way throughout the rest of the pregnancy. Well, that instruction resonated with me, and I'm sure it will resonate with you as an expectant father as well.

After calling the hospital to find out what was going to happen, it occurred to me that I would be spending a lot of time with the practitioner as well. As a result, I had to be satisfied with the final decisions. These were some of the key people in the process of discovering things for myself.

A Need for a Private Obstetrician, Doctor, or Midwife

Now, let me tell you something: if your partner is twenty, she should have been seeing a gynecologist for a few years. And, given that many gynecologists also practice obstetrics, it should come as no surprise that we had to have a woman's usual obstetrician/gynecologist (OB/GYN) deliver the baby.

Our obstetrician was rather pricey, but we weren't put off because our insurance company covered most of the bill, so keep your insurance company updated at frequent intervals.

One thing I noticed about our private obstetrician was that she wasn't really private. Mrs. Adams, our obstetrician/gynecologist, did have several cases. So, it came as no surprise to me that she wasn't the doctor present during the delivery. But here's the thing: these kinds of things don't always happen; it's sort of 'chance stuff,' she may attend the birth, or she may not, depending on the schedule on the day of the birth.

But there is no method to avoid this, as you cannot ensure that your usual doctor is not scheduled to see someone or another patient on the day of labor, unless your labor is planned, or you have a scheduled c-section.

In our case, no matter how hard we tried to reach her on the deal day, she was extremely busy. So, we had to adapt—don't worry, we'll go through this in greater depth in the following chapter.

The nurse who spoke to us on the initial day said that my doctor most likely wouldn't be able to attend. She said the doctor already had a full patient schedule for the day, but there was another well qualified doctor that would be available. The nurse explained that this wasn't unusual. Physicians were generally busy seeing many patients throughout the day. That still bothered me as a man and a parent, but I understood and had to accept it because I wasn't the only one with a pregnant wife. I texted the doctor directly, and her response was, "I'll try my best to be there"—that was all she said.

However, my wife wanted an obstetrician because she couldn't handle the pain of childbirth, and I understood.

Sandra Howell-White discovered that women who perceive delivery as risky, or who want to have a voice in regulating their pain or the length of their labor, tend to choose obstetricians.

What about your Family physician and Mid-wives?

I'm sure many of you are wondering about this by now. As I found during the process, while many family physicians provide obstetrical care, not all of them do. So, my wife and I checked with ours to see whether he did, and it was not the case. If you're okay with that and your partner is fine with childbirth, then go ahead and start the process.

We had a family doctor, and he had counseled us on what to do based on my wife's past childbirths and how he saw this one now.

He constantly told me, "I don't want to take any chances."

And I completely understood. I like how many physicians are dedicated to their professions and treat their patients as if they were their own family.

But when it came to our family physician, one of the major benefits we received from him was that he frequently showed concern and checked in, making random checks to see whether the mother and the baby were well. In essence, the circumstance that frequently occurs—dashing from one doctor to another—was eventually reduced, and it was a breath of fresh air to me whenever I saw him outside my door to check on my wife.

So, what distinguishes these family doctors from average care? Some of you may have one, but for those who do not, keep in mind that, like other doctors, family physicians are typically in group practices, and there is no guarantee that the doctor you know will be on call the day your baby is born. So, if possible, you can contact the other doctors in the practice, as well as any OB/GYN your family doctor may work with.

Moreover, most of these family doctors or FPs do not do cesarean sections or assisted deliveries, so they will require an OB/GYN backup. Make sure you're familiar with this individual because he or she may be in charge of the delivery if things get tough or problematic.

Midwives were another option that my wife and I discussed. And this was a proposal given by my mother-in-law when we decided to conceive our first kid.

Midwives, in my humble view, are becoming increasingly popular in the United States, despite the fact that they are not as widespread in Europe or other areas of the world. And we were ready to bring one into the process, when we changed our minds for personal reasons, namely our finances. However, if you like the notion, you may wish to include one in the process, even if your spouse has a conventional OB or obstetrician.

According to the researcher, Howell-White, women who expect their spouses to be actively involved in labor and delivery and who place a high importance on learning about the birth process are far more likely to choose a midwife. Surprisingly, women with no commitment or who have never employed a midwife are also included.

Certified nurse-midwives (CNMs) are licensed nurses who have completed two or three years of extra obstetrics training and passed the specific certification examinations. They can give birth in hospitals, birth facilities, or even at home. However, because their training is frequently in simple, low-risk deliveries, CNMs must collaborate closely with a physician in case an issue arises.

Some states in the United States have introduced a new title; certified midwife (CM), which is stated to allow practitioners who are not nurses but who go through the same training and complete the same examinations as CNMs to function as midwives.

As a result, many regular OB/GYN practices now include a CNM or, in certain circumstances, a CM on staff, recognizing that some of their patients may desire a midwife present for the delivery. Officially, your spouse is still under the care of the physician, whose services are covered by insurance, but she will still receive the more customized treatment she desires. However, keep in mind that because midwives are not doctors, they cannot conduct surgery and can only treat low-risk cases. Hopefully, none of these constraints will be an issue for you.

With that out of the way, if you are considering using a CNM or CM and need some assistance, all you need to do is contact the American College of Nurse-Midwives, or if you are not based in the United States, contact regular medical professionals in your country to give you some information, or you can check online as there are vast resources there.

And, according to my observations, there are numerous midwives who are neither certified nor licensed. Lay midwives are known to have extensive experience working with pregnant women and may even have specific training. However, they are not regulated and may not have completed any specialized midwife examinations, which simply means that they are not qualified to practice in hospitals or birthing facilities but solely in home settings.

Lay midwives, like CNMs or CMs, must collaborate with a doctor in the event of an emergency or a severe situation that they cannot handle.

BACK TO MY EXPERIENCES

When my wife and I eventually decided that we needed the OB/GYN, we were told to ask appropriate questions and acquire satisfactory answers, as we had in the past. You must ensure that the OB/GYN understands what he is about to do in order to avoid "sorry notes" or blunders later in the process.

We'd arranged a fifteen-minute appointment with our OB/GYN at that time. When asking questions, be specific and give honest and detailed responses about your wife and how you want the OB/GYN to handle the matter.

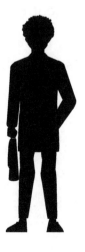

Here are some of the questions we asked our OB/GYNs

- Where do you deliver?

- Do you enable the mother and father to cut the umbilical cord?

- Do you normally hand the bare infant to the mother?

- Do you suction the infant or use forceps during delivery?

- How do you feel about a father aiding with childbirth?

- How do you feel about the mother taking the baby out of herself if she so desires?

- What type of monitoring do you recommend?

- What is your definition of a "high-risk" pregnancy?

- Do you allow dads to attend cesarean sections? If so, where do they stand (up by the woman's shoulders or down at the "business end")?

- What is your c-section rate, and how do you decide whether to proceed with the surgery?

- How do you feel about cesareans, labor inductions, and episiotomies?

- Where do you stand on the natural vs. medicated debate?

- Do you do amniocentesis yourself?

- What percentage of your patients' newborns do you deliver? What are your contingency plans if you are unable to attend?

- Are you board certified? Do you have any specialties or training?

- Do you have any recommendations for special birth preparation methods?

- How do you feel about the father being there for prenatal tests and the delivery? Are you excited about it or merely tolerant of it?

Questions for Midwives

- Are you licensed or certified? And by which organization?

- How many babies have you delivered?

- How do you decide whether to move the patient to a hospital or to the care of a physician? How often does that happen?

- What is the most common position taken by your patients during labor and for the delivery? (This helps to certify whether or not the midwife understands what he or she is doing and how he or she may contribute to a safe birth.)

- What is the function of the physician in your practice?

- How frequently does a physician become involved in the treatment of patients?

- With which doctors and hospitals do you work?

Questions for both OB/GYNs and Midwives

- How much experience do you have with twins or more? (This is a crucial question if you and/or your spouse have a family history of multiple births, believe that your partner is carrying more than one child, or have had the appropriate scan to find out.)

- Can women walk, move, and shower during the early stages of labor? Can the infant be breastfed right after birth?

- How many sonograms (ultrasounds) do you typically recommend?

- What tests do you often prescribe for women like your spouse (based on her age, ethnicity, medical history, and risk factors)?

- Which prenatal tests do you recommend? Which do you require?

- Are you willing to wait until the umbilical cord has stopped pulsing before clamping it?

- What and who is permitted in the delivery room (apart from you, Dad—friends, relatives, cameras, webcams, etc.)?

- Will you come in if labor starts when you are not on call?

- What is your definition of "high risk?"

- What proportion of your patients had natural, unmedicated deliveries in the previous year?

- What insurance, if any, do you accept?

- What are your pricing and payment plans?

- Do you have a helpline we may call if we are worried about something?

After all the necessary questions, we then came to the **Bills.**

Let me warn you right now that having a baby isn't inexpensive. How much you must come up with will depend on how and where your child is delivered, as well as which of the endless permutations of deductible, coinsurance, copays, and out-of-pocket maximums you have.

And, according to the Agency for Healthcare Research and Quality in the United States, which is part of the United States Department of Health and Human Services, the average rate for vaginal birth is just under $9000, which is about quadruple what it was in the 1990s. And the average cesarean fee is about $16,000, which is 2.5 times what it was in the mid-1990s.

In my instance, private insurance paid an average of sixty-six percent of my wife's prenatal expenditures, and seventy percent of the birth charges.

However, according to further agency estimates, private insurance paid at least eighty percent of prenatal care costs and eighty-eight percent of delivery costs. But the thing is, even if you have decent insurance, twelve to twenty percent may quickly add up. Keep in mind though that what the practitioner receives is nearly often far less than the standard sticker—so it all relies, possibly, on your luck.

In the part that follows, you'll get an idea of the costs for a normal and not-so-typical pregnancy and birthing experience, broken down in how it affected me and what is typical, though prices may change in the future for fathers and others reading this.

In addition, it is a good idea to review your insurance

coverage, determine how much it will cover, and begin planning how you will pay for the rest of it right away.

This also covers any fees you may have spent for fertility testing and treatment.

What I'm referring to here are the expenses I incurred when my wife became pregnant. Even if you are adopting, creating a budget is essential.

Pregnancy and Childbirth Fees

Most doctors will charge a set cost for the partner's treatment throughout the pregnancy. This often includes monthly appointments throughout the first two trimesters, biweekly visits for the following month or so, then weekly visits until birth.

But don't make the mistake of believing that's all you have to pay. I made the same error, which is why I'm warning you about what most of us decide in the end. Bills for blood and urine tests, ultrasounds, hospital expenses, and other treatments will almost certainly arrive in your mailbox at least once a month. Here are some of the things my wife and I had to decide on and pay for in order to have our baby. And I include some that you might be interested in, such as midwifery; don't worry, I'll explain what you'll need to pay for in this respect.

OB/GYN

In this regard, we paid around $3,500, and when I inquired further, I was told that it usually ranges between 2,500 and $6,500 for regular prenatal care and a problem-free vaginal birth. If your physicians determines that your wife will require a C-section to deliver the baby, you'll need to spend a few thousand extra dollars. In my instance, my doctor met with me to go through my charges and the services he provided.

Furthermore, I propose that you discuss which insurance plans, if any, you have. Inquire with the doctor about your insurance coverage. You should also inquire whether they will bill your insurance company directly or require a deposit. Most of them want to get around twenty-five percent of the projected amount in advance, whether you may pay in installments, or they demand their charge to be paid in whole before delivery.

Midwife

The typical cost of a midwife-assisted birth is $2000 to $4000, although this can vary widely depending on where you live and whether you expect her to stay with you throughout labor or only the time up until the doctor takes over for the delivery. If you are delivering at home, you will need to include in the cost of the materials that the midwife believes you will require for the delivery, such as bandages, sterile pads, and other items.

Lab and Other Costs

- Ultrasound; this might cost up to $250 per visit. In a typical pregnancy, you do not need to spend as much money. In most situations of pregnancy, this necessitates more than one.

- Blood: You should budget at least $200 to $1,500 for various blood tests during your pregnancy. I paid $200; yours may differ.

Then it came to our **prenatal testing.**

My wife was a candidate for a prenatal test or amniocentesis, and we were supposed to spend 1050 dollars. And, according to my research, the bill for these run from $1,000 to $1,500.

I could almost feel my wife keeping it in, tenderly massaging that bundle of pleasure in her tummy. I was right by her, giving her all the help, she needed as I looked about and compared the costs with each step we took. It was also enjoyable, but I despised the hospital's sterile odor, which I had to accept in order to not add to my wife's discomfort.

In summary, you should avoid agitating your spouse during situations like these since doing so might be harmful to the child. So, make sure you constantly talk to her about pleasurable things, and if there is an emergency on the side, you will need to consider waiting to share until she has given birth and slept for at least a week.

As we handled the other bills, we went to the genetic counselling unit, which we had done in the past with other hospitals, but if you are at a new hospital, they will still want to conduct the procedure, so don't assume anything. Even in our hospital, they had to check their system to see if they were aware of our genetic testing before allowing us to leave. Genetic testing might cost between $400 and $800.

The nicest part was that when I wanted to find out the gender of my child on Wednesday, June 6, 2021, this is how it went.

"So, you're done with all of the tests for the time being," the doctor stated. "But we have one test and want to know whether you're interested."

I looked at my wife, who was also intrigued. "What do you mean, Doc?" I inquired.

"Well, do you wish to know the child's gender?" he asked.

My wife smiled, a little tight, but she held it together like the courageous lady she is. "I told him it's a girl," she grinned. "I can feel her kicking in me."

"No, it isn't; I told her it was a boy," I replied, and we all chuckled.

"Well, we'd have to resolve the dispute here," he remarked. "Would you prefer to have prenatal testing again but this time to determine the gender of the child?"

My wife agreed. "We really do," she said, smiling at me.

"Yes, and that would also be quite useful," the doctor remarked. "I know you've been doing your prenatal tests, but we need to check in often to see how the baby is doing in there."

We all agreed and went forward with it. We discovered it was a boy that day, so I won!

Lesson

- Many hospitals now offer their own birth rooms, or even birthing facilities, where the patient's sole purpose is to bring someone into the world.

- If your partner is considered "high risk," (she's carrying twins or more, is over 35, has had complications in the past, especially during delivery, has any medical risk factors, or was told anything that might be of concern by her practitioner), then a hospital birth should be the only option here.

Chapter

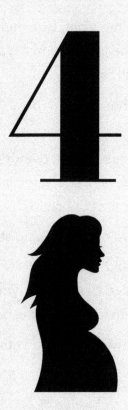

4

THE HOSPITAL, THE MOTHER WHO SUSPECTS

My wife began to feel dizzy and vomited a few days later. I felt something had gone wrong and had to take her to the hospital to check.

I was frantically packing items that day, baby diapers and other necessities, because I felt it was the baby's way of expressing it wanted to be born. I came downstairs all stuffed in arms as soon as I finished packing everything I needed.

"What are you doing?" my wife said as she sat on the sofa with her legs apart.

"I'm packing some stuff for the baby," I explained. "Perhaps now is the moment."

She smirked and thrust her arm forward as she attempted to stand. That was a sign that I should help her, which I did right away. When you observe a woman in this posture, you must gently raise her up. This is because the weight of the baby is too much and her center hinge is restricted, making it difficult for a woman to stand up comfortably.

"We don't really need it," she added as she led the way to the door.

I was perplexed. All of the vomiting and early morning headaches were supposed to be signs of this.

"But isn't it supposed to be an indication that the baby is about to come out?" I enquired.

She shook her head. "No," she said as she continued to walk to the door.

"Not all infants are the same," she said dryly before exiting.

That struck a chord with me. "Not all infants are the same," so the reactions you might observe when giving birth to a first born may differ from what you'll notice while giving birth to a second since all kids have their own manner of coming into this world.

We were at the hospital a few minutes later—another thing I want to mention is that before the baby is due, make sure you have planned a clear route to the hospital and your transportation is in good working order prior to the birth.

Now, in continuation of all the bills we paid in that hospital:

- We'd paid for a problem-free vaginal delivery and a twenty-four-hour hospital stay, which cost between $4,500 and $9000. It all depends on where you reside.

- If you intend to spend the night in the hospital with your spouse, you need to add $250 each day.

- I also realized that, while many people are concerned about preterm birth, there is also the issue of late delivery. If your child decides to stay inside for more than seven to ten days over his due date, your spouse may need to have labor induced, which can cost between $1,000 and $3,000.

- Then there's the anesthesiologist, whose salary ranges from $1,000 to $1,500, depending on what they do and how much time they spend doing it.

- If your spouse gives birth prematurely, within a few weeks, and your infant requires special care, the bills— the majority of which you will ideally never see—can be in the hundreds of thousands!

So that's all I had to pay before or on the day we went to the hospital. This is why I stated it isn't a cheap thing to do. The average cost of a vaginal birth is around $2,900 (with insurance), and up to $19,000 (without insurance). We will later discuss purchasing baby food, diapers, wife's meals, and many other topics in detail in this book.

What if your spouse needs a C-section? What are the chances and how much will it cost?

The first thing you should know is that this is not an uncommon thing. About thirty percent of women have c-sections, so don't be surprised if your doctor agrees. Furthermore, even though it is common, it is still considered major surgery and is costly. The procedure that the OB/GYN will do is not included in his or her fixed charge. You will also have to pay for at least two more physicians to help you, as well as a nurse who must be there to care for the infant.

A C-section requires a lengthier hospital stay, generally four to five days, as well as more nurse care, bandages, pain medicine, and all other supplies.

If the baby is healthy, you can probably take him or her home while your partner stays. But chances are you'll want the baby to stay with your spouse, especially if she's nursing. The baby's additional time in the nursery is also much more expensive.

Another piece of advice or heads up I'd want to provide you is to **double-check the list of items or bills** the hospital sends you.

My partner and I double-checked our birth-related costs. We did this because we know hospitals are operated by humans, and humans are prone to making mistakes. In fact, according to one research conducted by Equifax, nine out of ten hospital invoices contain errors, and they are rarely in your favor.

As we went through, we were careful to search for double-billings, services that we never received, maybe a private room when we were actually sharing one, brand name meds when we only got generics, and any other odd lingo that we encountered.

We also had to keep a watch on operations that never happened. And this might be due to my wife's rapid observations at the moment. My wife has heard stories about new parents being charged for their baby's circumcision that didn't even happen.

Some of these double-charged items may appear little, but they may quickly add up, especially if you are footing a large share of the tab. According to the Equifax report, the average inaccuracy was over $1300. According to collaborative research conducted by Harvard's Medical and Law Schools, "almost half of all Americans who file for bankruptcy do so due to medical bills." Around ten percent of those were connected to delivery.

Even if my insurance covered all our costs, examining them was a must. And, while most insurance companies have their own internal auditors, they will only be able to catch expenses that are above "the normal and customary" or treatments that are simply not covered.

The important point to remember here is that some of these insurance companies may only cover certain items. So, read your policy carefully, and if you have any issues, contact your agent or one of the company's underwriters.

While reading your insurance coverage, keep the following in mind:

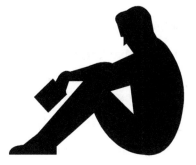

- How long before the delivery must the insurer be notified of the pregnancy and projected due date? Noncompliance with the carrier's instructions may easily result in a reduction in the amount they will pay for the pregnancy—and this was about to happen to me if I didn't act soon.

- When may the infant be added to the policy? All pregnancy and birth-related expenditures will be billed to your partner until the baby is born.

After the delivery, however, your spouse and the new baby will receive separate bills, and all baby-related expenditures, such as medicine, diapers, blankets, and many other baby products, as well as hospital charges, will be billed to the baby.

Some carriers require you to add the baby to your policy as early as thirty days before the delivery, while most let you wait until thirty days after the birth. Again, failure to properly follow the insurer's guidelines might result in a reduction in coverage.

Now, if the worst happens, hospital emergency rooms are required by federal law to provide your spouse with an initial examination and any necessary emergency care, even if you cannot afford to pay. But it is no alternative for the type of regular prenatal care that will assure a good pregnancy, a healthy baby, and a healthy mother.

So, whether you are insured, uninsured or you just need assistance paying for the prenatal care your spouse needs. Then your first step would be to search online for all essential Medicare or Medicaid benefits that your partner is entitled for. You shouldn't feel terrible if you fall into this group. Medicaid covers around forty percent of maternal hospitalizations connected to delivery. Because these benefits differ by state, you should also consult your state's health agency.

If you choose the low-cost alternatives and reside in a city with a big teaching hospital, your spouse may be able to get prenatal care at the hospital's obstetrical clinic. If this is the case, you will spend far less than you would for a private physician.

The one disadvantage is that your baby will almost probably be delivered by an inexperienced—yet highly supervised—doctor or medical student. This is not to say that you would not receive high-quality treatment. Clinics are frequently outfitted with cutting-edge technology, and the young professionals who staff them are taught all of the latest techniques by some of the top professors in the country.

MORNING SICKNESS CONTINUES

My gorgeous wife's morning sickness lingered, but the last time we went to the hospital after paying all the necessary fees, the doctor told us not to worry and that all my wife needed to do was eat a good diet. It astounded me that all of my wife's dizziness and headaches were caused by a lack of sufficient nourishment (after the doctor kept harping on it, telling us that's what the baby wanted). We had no choice but to heed our doctor, who had given us a deadline and instructed us to emphasize salad days.

The doctor provided us the list of items that were vital to my wife's health and fetal growth, even though it was long overdue at this time.

- Fruits: Cantaloupe, honeydew, prunes, oranges (my wife adores oranges), and red or pink grapefruit

- Vegetables: carrots, red sweet peppers, pumpkins, spinach, sweet potatoes, tomatoes, and cooked greens.

- Proteins: lamb and pig, sardines and pollock, herring, trout, nuts and seeds, lean meat.

- Grains: Cooked cereals with folic acid and iron were required.

- Dairy: Soymilk, skim or 1 percent milk, fat-free or low-fat yogurt.

- Frozen smoked seafood.

- Frozen meat spreads and pate.

- Raw and undercooked seafood, eggs, and meat. No raw fish sushi for her, but cooked sushi was fine.

- Hot dogs and luncheon meats, unless boiled till boiling hot before serving, were provided to my wife, who enjoyed it.

- Unpasteurized milk and meals manufactured with

unpasteurized milk, such as soft cheeses like fresco, queso blanco, Camembert brie, or blue-veined cheeses, were not permitted. Only if they were labeled with pasteurized milk.

Now, if you want to prepare something for her, make sure you follow these rigorous criteria: when handling and cooking food, observe these general food safety principles.

1. Wash your hands: Yes, whenever I was in the kitchen making my wife's meals. Before eating, chopping, or preparing, I took care to properly clean my hands as well as any raw vegetables under running tap water.

2. Clean: After handling and preparing raw foods, ensure sure all tools, such as counters and cutting boards, are sparkling clean.

3. Cook: Cook beef, pork, or poultry to a safe internal temperature as measured by a food thermometer.

4. Chill: Freeze any perishable items immediately.

Our doctor also advised us of the need of folic acid. The US Public Health Service recommends 400 micrograms (0.4 mg) of folic acid per day for all women of reproductive age. Folic acid is a vitamin that is found in:

- Nutritional supplements.
- Certain green leafy vegetables, as well as most nuts, berries, beans, citrus fruits, and fortified morning cereals.

Folic acid is almost essential because it helps lower the likelihood of neural tube abnormalities, which are birth disorders of the brain and spinal cord. Neural tube abnormalities can cause paralysis, incontinence, and even intellectual incapacity.

This brings back memories of how my wife would always request a certain salad she preferred. She would always crave it, so, men, be prepared, especially if your wife is constantly crying or pestering you. This doesn't imply she'll change her personality or turn you into a nanny overnight–far from it. Her taste buds and stomach secretions are just begging for a change of food, and this is in agreement with the baby's hunger.

Folic acid is especially useful in the first twenty-eight days after conception. The majority of neural tube defects occur at this stage. Unfortunately, some men may not even realize their wife is pregnant until after twenty-eight days. Folic acid supplementation should thus begin before conception and continue throughout pregnancy. The doctor or midwife would be the one to recommend the proper dose of folic acid to meet specific needs.

Women who use anti-epileptic medications, for example, may need to take more folic acid to avoid neural tube abnormalities. When considering or deciding to bring someone into the world, they should consult with their doctor.

Let's speak about the signs I noticed with my wife that made me nervous and may be occurring to you now or will happen to you when she gets pregnant.

Physically, you can see:

- Fuller breasts. Yes, my wife's breasts became bigger.

- Tiredness. She was exhausted most of the time, and I had to assist her with a variety of tasks.

- Dizziness. She often was dizzy at different stages in the pregnancy.

- Food cravings or aversions.

- As well as the typical symptoms of morning sickness, including nausea, vomiting, and heartburn.

Emotionally:

- My wife experienced mood swings and uncontrollable sobbing.

- Concern about the next nine months.

- A heightened sense of neediness or some sort of connection to you.

- Excited, stunned, a bit scared, or perhaps entirely depressed.

So, if you see any of these signs, don't panic. The infant is okay.

Chapter

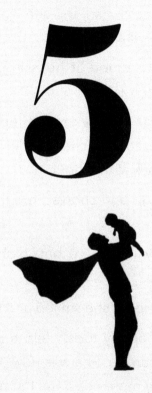

5

HOW I FELT WHEN SHE NOTIFIED ME SHE WAS PREGNANT

I remember the day like it was yesterday, I was in the bathroom taking a shower, and she kept calling me.

I came out of the water, ready to dry off. She was on the bed, giggling from ear to ear. I was astonished, thinking it was exciting news.

"What's going on?" I questioned, a little anxious, but still smiling as I went to my closet, turning back to see her gorgeous face.

"I want you to guess, darling," she whispered, her thighs clasped tightly as she stared.

"You know I'm not good at guessing, babe" I said. "So, please tell me what this is all about."

To be honest, I was already getting impatient. I had a lot of things to do that day, and her cheerful demeanor was the only thing holding me back at that hour.

She gently rose up and showed me the pregnancy stick. "This!" she shouted.

My mind instantly went there, but I didn't want to accept it, so I asked her, "What?"

"I'm pregnant, stupid," she smiled and hugged me.

I recall standing on my toes. I felt terrified, wondering if this was actually occurring. She was now expecting. We were now expecting to be more accurate. I turned to face her and grinned. "So, what's next?" I inquired.

"Well, the regular," she murmured, still clutching me and gazing at me with her head on my chest.

That day, I was getting ready to go to work, but I had to wait a bit to take in this bundle of news, which was a delight to me at the time.

I was thrilled she informed me, and joyfully carried her about the room, twirling her in delight.

So, when it comes to this sort of circumstance, there is no reason to be afraid or concerned about what may or may not occur.

I took the pregnancy stick (a small testing kit) and glanced at it again—we were both seated on the bed now. I will admit, the positive pregnancy test result made me very excited, but a little anxious as well. Overall, I knew things would work out how they're supposed to. My child was on his way into the world, and all I had to do was be prepared.

IRRATIONAL FEARS

After the initial euphoria wears off, a surprising number of men develop an unfounded worry that the child their spouse is carrying is not theirs. Psychologist Jerrold Lee Shapiro questioned over two hundred men whose partners were pregnant and discovered that sixty percent "acknowledged brief ideas, fantasies, or persistent suspicions that they might not be the biological father." The majority of these males do not believe their partners are having affairs. Rather, as researcher Shapiro explains, these thoughts are just indicators of a widespread sort of insecurity: the concern that many men have that they are incapable of achieving anything as extraordinary as producing life and that someone more capable must have done it. Most guys get over these sentiments fast, and most of the time it is once they see the child.

IVF fathers, who did not participate in the biological creation, have their own set of unreasonable anxieties. Many men are concerned that the sperm samples have been exchanged and that they will have a child of a different race. Actually, the issue isn't so much about race as it is about physical similarities. Most IVF couples do not feel compelled to reveal the details of their pregnancy. And, like any other father, they want their children to look like them—at least enough to avoid the usual "Oh my, the kid doesn't look anything like you" comments. They may decide to tell the children the genuine tale of their birth later on.

MORNING SICKNESS

Morning sickness affects between half and ninety percent of all pregnant women. Despite the catchy moniker, nausea, heartburn, and vomiting can hit at any time of day. Nobody knows what causes morning sickness. Some believe it is the pregnant woman's reaction to altering hormone levels, namely human chorionic gonadotropin (HCG), which is generated by the placenta and is detected by home pregnancy kits.

Others believe and argue that morning sickness is the body's natural way of protecting the developing baby from teratogens (toxins that cause birth abnormalities) and abortifacients (toxins that induce miscarriages). Morning sickness appears to go hand in hand with dietary aversions, which the vast majority of pregnant women suffer. Eggs, chicken, and fish are the most prevalent dietary aversions among pregnant women, as they deteriorate rapidly and might spread disease.

Morning sickness, whatever the source, usually goes away by the third month for most women. Until then, here are a few ways to assist your spouse. Although I've mentioned dietary aspects, let's talk about the day-to-day odd stuff that has to be done.

- Assist her in maintaining a high-protein, high-carbohydrate diet.

- Always offer her positive news. Morning sickness may sometimes be a godsend. Women who suffer severe morning sickness are less likely to miscarry, deliver prematurely, or have kids with low birth weight. According to some studies, the more severe the symptoms, the higher the baby's IQ. Knowing this is unlikely to help your spouse feel better. But it could always offer her something to grin about while she's bending over the toilet bowl—so tell her this and lift her spirits a little.

- Be aware that she needs plenty of rest and encourage her to get it.

- Investigate alternate therapies. Wristbands that push on the inside of the wrist have helped some women's symptoms, as has eating or drinking ginger. Furthermore, some studies suggests that inhaling peppermint oil and isopropyl alcohol can help lessen the length of symptoms. However, you must still consult with your practitioner before smelling, ingesting, or pushing on anything.

- Keep some pretzels, crackers, or rice cakes beside the bed—she'll need something to start and end the day with, and these are low in fat and calories and simple to digest.

- Make sure she takes her prenatal vitamins with food if her doctor advises her to. The doctor may also advise her to take extra vitamins B and K. For some women, prenatal supplements may aggravate morning sickness. Lissa Rankin frequently converts her patients to a chewable vitamin. If that fails, she just discontinues the vitamins for a few months. She frequently asserts that staying hydrated and consuming nutrition is more essential than taking vitamins.

- Go for a walk. Some women do find that exercises reduce nausea.

- Encourage her to eat small meals often throughout the day—every two hours if possible—and to eat before she feels dizzy or nauseated again. Rice and yogurt are particularly beneficial since they are less prone to produce nausea than fatty meals.

- Be aware of the sights and odors that make her uneasy and keep them away from her. Fatty or spicy meals are common offenders.

- Encourage her to drink plenty of fluids. You should also have a big water bottle close to the bed. Caffeine should be avoided at this time since it is more dehydrating. She could also wish to start the day with a modest amount of non-acidic juices like grape, apple, or flat Coke. The sweet flavor will encourage her to drink a bit more than she would normally.

HOW I STAYED INVOLVED

My wife and I worked out frequently, so if your partner was already working out before the pregnancy, she definitely won't need any more motivation to exercise. And, if her doctor allows, she may resume her usual exercise program and perform pretty much any type of workout she wants.

However, be aware that certain fitness clubs, for fear of being sued, may require a pregnant woman to provide a note from her doctor. If your partner was not physically active before the pregnancy, now is not the time for her to start rock climbing or training to climb higher peaks on a mountain. That doesn't imply she should spend her entire pregnancy on the couch. Exercise is crucial. It will aid in circulation and keep her energy levels up.

When my wife and I exercised together during her pregnancy, it helped keep her weight stable and appropriate. When we were completing the exercises together, I observed that it helped boost her mood and alleviate some of the regular pregnancy-related discomforts. It also enhanced her strength and endurance, both of which are helpful during birth.

Researchers James Clapp and Elizabeth Noble discovered that pregnant women who exercise had shorter labors and have healthier newborns. Others have discovered that exercise may reduce the likelihood that your spouse may deliver early or require a C-section.

However, because pregnancy may make even the fittest woman feel run down, she may not always feel like working out. This was pretty interesting to us; my wife had drastically lowered the rate at which she worked out. Nonetheless, working out alongside her might assist in inspiring her to do the activities she is comfortable performing. Don't make her do everything by herself. The most essential thing is to start slowly and push her if you see she's getting weary or exhausted. If your budget does not allow you to join a gym or a health club, you can always go on YouTube, subscribe to your favorite channels, and join your favorite pregnancy health clubs—there are many resources available online these days.

Whatever you choose, remember that you and your partner will benefit the most and have the least likelihood of damage if you exercise consistently, but don't force it. Thirty minutes on as many days as you can rather than irregularly. Here are some terrific ways to exercise together:

1. You can play tennis or gulf.

2. You can cycle.

3. You can weight lift if you are both capable of doing so.

4. You can swim, perform water aerobics, or snorkel.

5. You can perform low-impact aerobics or use low-impact exercise machines.

6. You can run, but make sure both of your knees favor it; get good shoes and run on soft surfaces.

7. You can do some yoga. But please, you will need to avoid the extreme stretches. This can cause damage to your partner's connective tissues, which are somewhat weakened during pregnancy.

8. Walking. It doesn't matter whether it is fast or slow, through your neighborhood, on a trail, or on a treadmill.

Before beginning any type of exercise regimen, consult with your practitioner or doctor and obtain his or her consent. If you are doing anything that may cause you to sweat, make sure to drink enough water. You should each drink a glass or two an hour before you begin, followed by another four to eight ounces every fifteen to twenty minutes while working out.

The Don'ts When Working Out

Some of the sports I talk about were ones my wife wanted to do while she was still pregnant. To be honest, I was horrified when she proposed doing such strenuous workouts while our child was still inside her.

1. **Downhill skiing**: Do not do so unless you are an expert. And even if you do want to do it, you must tread carefully. Yes, my wife skied, but she avoided the difficult runs, where you risk a major fall.

2. **Heavy lifting**: This might place undue strain on the internal organs.

3. **High-impact sports**: I've spoken with a lot of OB/GYNs over the years, and I've yet to find one who believes that merely falling causes a miscarriage, especially in the first trimester. However, very abrupt impacts, such as vehicle accidents, can sometimes induce a miscarriage due to the quick shock from mother to child. As a result, it's a good idea to minimize or avoid high-contact sports like roller derby, hockey, and boxing.

4. **Hot tubs/steam baths and saunas**: It is better to avoid anything that might elevate your partner's body temperature above 39 degrees Celsius. To cool itself, the body transfers blood away from internal organs–including the uterus and the fetus–and toward the skin.

5. **Overheating**: Your companion should not overdress and should keep her exercises to a minimum. I constantly encouraged my wife to take several pauses anytime we were both doing something strenuous, and I always told her to drink plenty of water before, during, and after the activity.

6. **Overdoing i**t: If she can't hold a regular conversation while exercising, she's working too hard; stop her!

7. **Any sport that is extreme**: Please avoid horseback riding, in-line skiing, ice skating, and, beginning around the seventh month, biking. Taking a tumble while participating in one of these sports might be risky for a non-pregnant person. The hazards are especially larger for someone who struggles with balance.

My final piece of advice is to not panic if your partner did any of these things before you found out she was pregnant. To begin with, there is nothing you can do about it right now and tormenting yourself won't help. Second, the chances are small that whatever she did before she discovered she was pregnant would have had a negative influence on the fetus. All you have to do now is be cautious till the baby is born.

Lesson

- A pregnant woman should and can exercise but avoid high-impact activities.

- Don't be alarmed about morning sickness; it's normal.

Chapter

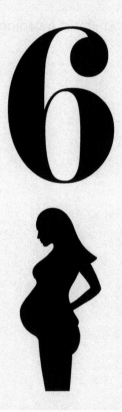

6

WHAT SHOULD SHE EAT?

The notion of healthy nutrition hasn't changed much since you learned about the food pyramid or, if you prefer, the four fundamental food categories in sixth grade. However, now that you have a pregnant spouse, she will require around three hundred more calories per day than before. And if she was underweight, she'd need a bit more that that—in this case, you'll need to consult a doctor.

If she was overweight before becoming pregnant, now is not the time to start a diet. At the same time, the fact that she is 'eating for two' does not give her license to eat whatever she wants. Her practitioner will undoubtedly recommend a diet for your partner to follow, but there are a few nutritional basics to keep in mind at all times.

My wife and I were interested in what she should nourish her body with.

Let's roughly go through all of the nutrition she paid attention to, and perhaps yours would have to do the same.

Fatty Foods

Despite all the hype about low-or-no-fat diets, the fact is that your partner, like everyone else in the world, needs to consume at least some fat. She will probably be getting most of what she needs in the other things she eats during the day; however, fat should account for no more than thirty percent of her overall calorie intake. A diet high in fatty foods is not beneficial for her or your growing child. Monosaturated fats, such as olive oil, avocado, canola oil, and peanuts, are the best, followed by polysaturated fats, such as mayonnaise, margarine, and walnuts. Saturated fats, such as bacon, butter, lard, and trans fats, are the worst. Basically, anything with the phrases "partially hydrogenated" or "hydrogenated" on the ingredients list.

IRON

If your companion does not receive enough iron, she may become anemic and tired. In this instance, all she has to do is eat at least three servings of iron-rich meals every day. Dried fruits, spinach, lentils, meat, and fortified cereals are all rich sources of iron. However, because your pregnant wife's iron intake is being utilized to produce the fetus's blood, she may require more than she can acquire from food alone.

If such is the case, her doctor will probably prescribe some over-the-counter vitamins after the third month. The doctor may also advise her to take prenatal vitamins, which include additional iron. If feasible, your companion should take the pills with a glass of orange juice. If she takes it alongside vitamin C, it will assist her body absorb the iron. However, a word of caution is in order here: taking iron supplements may result in constipation.

PROTEIN

A typical lady needs forty-five grams of protein each day. And your pregnant lady should consume seventy to eighty grams every day. If she is pregnant with twins, she will need to boost her protein intake by another twenty to twenty-five grams per day, but not until the fourth or fifth month, when the fetus is eight weeks old and has at least 125,000 neurons. Then, by the end of the nineteenth week, there are more than twenty-five billion neurons, the most your child will ever have.

Many nutritionists feel that a high protein diet, particularly during the first nineteen weeks of pregnancy, promotes this increase in brain cell proliferation in the newborn. Fortunately, most women consume an adequate amount of protein, so you won't have to worry about this.

If you must supplement, lean proteins are always the best option. Low-fat milk is one of the simplest sources of protein, with around eight grams in one glass. Pregnant moms who drank four glasses of milk per day were less likely to have children who had multiple sclerosis than women who drank fewer than three glasses per month. If your companion is unable to consume milk, large doses of Vitamin D showed comparable outcomes.

However, before she takes any supplements, please consult with her doctor or practitioner. Skinless chicken, low-fat cheese, lean meats, tofu or soyabean curd, peanut butter, and fried fish are other excellent sources. The eggs must also be cooked, not raw—having hard boiled eggs on hand is very convenient and beneficial to the newborn.

WATER

My wife had to drink at least eight ounces of water, and the water had to be unsweetened and caffeine-free. If she was going to do a workout with me or was pregnant during the heat, she had to drink a lot of water. This will assist your spouse in restoring the water she loses when she perspires, which she will do more of during pregnancy, as well as move waste items out of her system. Keep in mind that almost half of the population is dehydrated at any one time, putting them at a higher risk of developing a variety of problems, including kidney stones and urinary tract malignancies.

Grains and other Complex carbohydrates

Grains, which include breads and cereals, are essentially

fuel for your partner's body, and she should consume at least four servings every day.

I made rice and curry soup for my wife, which was one of her favorite dishes. And because her body will burn the fuel first, if she doesn't get enough there may not be sufficient amounts for the baby. Grains are often low in calories and abundant in zinc, chromium, and magnesium, all of which are vital elements. They are also high in fiber, which will assist your spouse battle the constipating impact of iron supplements. Whole-grain breads are good sources; please avoid white bread for at least a few months, add instead brown rice, dried beans, quinoa, and raw potatoes, which are dietary pleasures she may enjoy during this period.

GREEN AND YELLOW VEGETABLES

Green and yellow veggies, which weirdly include mango and cantaloupe, are fantastic providers of vitamin A and B, which will assist your partner's body absorb all the additional protein she'll be eating.

Vitamin A may also help prevent bladder and kidney infections. Furthermore, these veggies are high in folic acid, which can help minimize the risk of brain and spinal cord problems, particularly in the early months of pregnancy. Your partner's prenatal vitamins will supplement the folic acid she gets from her diet. The deeper the green, the healthier it is for your partner; she should attempt to consume a serving or two every day. And, hey, it wouldn't hurt to do the same.

CALCIUM

Calcium is required for the formation of the baby's bones. And, because so much of your partner's calcium intake goes directly to the baby, she must make sure she gets plenty for herself.

My wife took at least 1,200 mg per day in the form of milk, thus your pregnant wife should take 1200 to 1500 mg every day. If not, the growing fetus will drain it from your partner's bones, thereby increasing her chance of getting osteoporosis later in life. Milk and other dairy products are the finest calcium sources. However, if your spouse is allergic to milk or lactose intolerant, a condition that affects around fifty million Americans, many physicians would urge her to avoid it, especially if she plans to breastfeed, because her milk allergy might be passed on to the baby. Alternate calcium sources include canned pink salmon with extremely soft bones, broccoli, tofu, calcium-fortified orange juice, oyster-shell calcium pills, eggs, and TUMS 500s.

CITRUS FRUIT AND OTHER FOODS HIGH IN VITAMIN C

Vitamin C is necessary for the body's production of collagen, which is the substance that keeps the tissue together. It also promotes the growth of the baby's bones and teeth. My wife enjoyed any fruit high in vitamin C; oranges were her favorite.

ORGANIC: WHAT'S THE CRAZE ABOUT IT?

You're in luck since grocery store aisles are brimming with organic options. But how much of this enthusiasm is a sham; simply another reason to mark things up even more? I don't have a precise figure, but it seems reasonable to strive to restrict the number of pesticides, antibiotics, hormones, and other unpleasant muck in our food.

The Environmental Agency agrees with the assessment that avoiding the worst tainted fruits and vegetables can cut your exposure by up to eighty percent. My wife and I have a tiny garden on which we can rely on occasion. If you don't have a small garden, you may purchase online, but make sure you purchase one hundred percent organic, grown with little or no pesticides or fertilizers.

Here are some organic items you will need to purchase:

- Spinach
- Cherries
- Bell
- Celery
- Peaches
- Apples
- Blueberries
- Nectarines
- Strawberries
- Peppers

There is no need to buy organic:

- Peas
- Asparagus
- Eggplant

- Mangos
- Sweet corn
- Avocado
- Onion
- Pineapple

THINGS THAT NEED TO BE WHOLLY AVOIDED

The stuff you need to know here is that if your partner does any of these, so does your baby.

1. **Caffeine:** Caffeine abstinence is critical in the early months. Some studies have found that pregnant women who consume more than 200-300 mg per day, or two or three good-sized cups of coffee, had a higher chance of miscarriage, early delivery, or having a low-birth weight baby than women who passed up on Starbucks and kept their money in their handbag. Caffeine-free drinks are the safest bet. If she truly wants coffee, limiting her to one cup per day should be enough. Check with the doctor for the ultimate word.

2. **Cigarettes:** When a pregnant woman inhales cigarette smoke, her womb fills with carbon monoxide, resins, tar, and nicotine, preventing oxygen and nutrition delivery to the fetus. Smoking by mothers raises the chance of low-birth-weight infants and miscarriage. There is also some evidence that paternal smoking or exposing your spouse and her child to secondhand smoke is just as harmful.

If you believe that being within your partner protects the baby from your smoke, or that smoking doesn't matter early in pregnancy, I must disappoint you. The simple line is that if you are a smoker, you must quit today. If she is, urge her to quit and assist her in any way you can. Surprisingly, many men put off quitting or urging their spouses to quit for fear of causing marital conflict. That is a poor decision. The potential threat to your baby surpasses the danger to your relationship, and e-cigarettes are no better. Although e-cigarettes reduce secondhand smoke, most of these products include nicotine, which is potentially toxic and addicting to your partner and baby. Many also include diethylene glycol, a highly dangerous chemical used in antifreeze, as well as nitrosamines, a carcinogen present in actual cigarettes.

3. **Insecticides, weed killers, and more**: As long as you're taking over the gardening, all you need to do now is put on your gloves and transport a load of chemical fertilizer and pesticides to the nearest toxic waste disposal facility. If your usual garbage collection service is aware of its presence, they will refuse to pick it up. Prolonged and recurrent exposure to these hazardous compounds has been associated with birth abnormalities. If you need pesticides and fertilizers, now is the time to go organic.

In addition, you must keep your spouse away from additional chemical pollutants, such as diazinon, a typical cockroach killer, as well as no-pest strips, flea sprays and collars, and pesticide bombs. DDE and PCBS have severe harmful impacts. When children are exposed to those chemicals in utero, they tend to be two inches taller and weigh more as teenagers than children who were not exposed, and they commonly begin puberty too early.

4. **Recreational drugs**: Avoid this during pregnancy. This is because unborn children might become addicted and there are many harmful side effects that transfer to the fetus, including risk of death. Also, a mother can be charged with abuse for using drugs during pregnancy and be incarcerated, losing custody of her child. If the father is found to be aware of her habit, he too can be charged.

5. **Hair Dyes**: Long-term usage of hair dyes by adults has been linked to an elevated risk of many forms of cancer. But wait a minute, might hair dyes be absorbed into a pregnant woman's scalp, enter the bloodstream, and damage the fetus? That one is up for discussion. Some people think that's fine since no one is going to drink it; she's just going to put it in her hair. While some disagree, they point to extensive evidence indicating that wearing hair color may impact a growing fetus on a cellular level and may raise a child's chance of reproductive and developmental issues. I'm not sure which is accurate, but why take the chance. The simplest option would be for your spouse to refrain from using hair color while pregnant—at the very least during the first three months while the baby's organs and nervous system are developing. If you can't persuade her that her hair looks good as it is, have her check online for less hazardous hair coloring.

6. **Cat feces:** Although cat feces have little nutritional value, they do contain a high concentration of the parasites found in uncooked foods. So, if you have a cat and want to be chivalrous, take over cleaning the litter box for the length of the pregnancy. Most ladies do not have a problem with litter boxes. She has a far higher chance of coming into touch with cat excrement while she is outdoors, digging the garden, which appears to many cats to be more of a larger litter box.

7. **Certain foods**: Toxoplasma gondii, a parasite found in cat feces, is present in raw meats and fish. This parasite blinds the fetus and affects the infant's nervous system. Unpasteurized milk and soft cheeses like Brie may contain a bacteria called Listeria. Salmonella, another parasite, may be present in raw eggs and chicken. My wife's first OB/GYN was Chinese, and she had no problem with her eating sushi, although other fish items require extreme caution. The FDA advises pregnant women to avoid exotic marine species such as shark, mackerel, and tilefish, as well as swordfish, since they may contain high amounts of mercury. Reduce your consumption of albacore tuna to one or two servings per week. If she likes fish or seafood, salmon, pollack, and shrimp are the greatest alternatives right now because they are low in mercury.

8. **Fasting**: Please do not allow her go with it until the doctor has approved it. Your spouse should never go twenty-four hours without eating anything, let alone only sipping a cup of water; this is extremely risky for

the fetus, regardless of religious affiliation or health organizations that tell you this is an ideal practice. This is especially critical during the first nineteen weeks of pregnancy, when the baby's brain is forming.

FOR THE VEGETARIANS

If your partner is a vegetarian, there's no reason she can't obtain enough nutrition to sustain the baby and herself, especially if she drinks milk and eats eggs. However, if she is a devout vegan, you should look online for vegan eggs and milk, or she may go to her practitioner, who can give her advice and possibly provide her some of the nutrients her diet may be lacking via pills or over-the-counter medications.

HUNGER

One thing I always underestimated was how hungry my wife was. During this time, I believed the adage "feeding for two." She'd get what she wanted and be done with the food in less than a second. Even if she had a snack before leaving the workplace, she'd be hungry by the time she arrived home.

We divided the tasks before the pregnancy, and I was doing a lot of the housework, so when she became pregnant, things didn't alter all that much at home. But there was one thing I wasn't very good at around the house, and it was my wife who took over, and that was cooking. Here are a few things that must be done to avoid this.

- When you're out with friends, keep some munchies in the glove compartment: Her energy levels might drop at any time, and a handful of almonds, raisins, or a granola bar can come in handy.

- Prepare a nutritious dinner for her: Allow her to enjoy a few extra precious moments in bed with her excellent meal in the morning. Pamper her during this time; I did, and it worked really well for me.

- Go grocery shopping; Even if your spouse still organizes meals and creates shopping lists. Going to the supermarket will save her an hour or so a week of walking around on floors that are difficult even for non-pregnant people's feet. Furthermore, many women who suffer from severe morning sickness discover that being at a grocery store, surrounded by so much food is simply too much for them to bear. If your spouse conducted the shopping before the pregnancy, ask her to write a specific list of the products she regularly bought.

- Do some meal planning: This simply means you'll need to spend some time reading decent cookbooks and seeking recipes that will not trigger her nausea. Make a list of the ingredients you'll need as you read. Although meal planning might not appear to be difficult, it is time demanding, especially when you consider the extra time you will have to spend at the grocery store.

- Learn to prepare basic, quick meals: There are several cookbooks that specialize in dishes that can be produced in less than thirty minutes. So, all you must do is go online and search Amazon, or you can go to YouTube and watch videos of people cooking the items you want to prepare step by step.

WHAT I NEEDED TO STOCK UP ON ANYTIME I HEADED TO THE GROCERY STORE

Anytime I was on my way to the grocery store, I always had a list of all I wanted to buy.

- Doughnuts
- Raisins and other dried fruits
- Frozen berries and grapes
- Fresh fruit
- Fresh vegetables that can be eaten raw, which includes cucumbers, celery, tomatoes and carrots.
- Crackers
- Bottled water
- Pure fruit Jams
- Natural peanut butter
- Fresh eggs and hard-boiled eggs
- Low-fat, naturally sweetened yogurt
- Nonfat cottage cheese
- Skim milk
- Whole-grain bread
- Tomato or vegetable juice
- Whole-wheat pasta
- Unsweetened cereals

THE FINAL THING YOU NEED TO TAKE NOTE OF

Throughout her pregnancy, I assisted my wife in eating well, even though she would gripe and say "No" when she didn't like a type of food. I was attentive. You must ensure that she is eating well so that she can have a healthy child.

And one thing I always kept in mind when serving my wife was to never be too rough on her. Never show her my worry, if I had one at the time, or how negative I was about certain things.

Being pregnant is difficult enough without having someone standing over her shoulder condemning every decision she makes. While she'd be better off eating just healthy meals all of the time, an odd order of fries or a candy bar won't harm her long-term health.

Finally, you must be supportive. This simply means that you should aim to eat as healthily as she does. If you really must have a banana split and do not intend to share it, do it on your own time and do not penalize her for it in her state.

Lesson

- When it comes to your pregnant wife, nutrition is of the utmost importance.

- Please pay close attention to the do's and don'ts in this chapter. (What she needs to consume, such as fatty meals and water, and what she does not need to take in or drink, such as cigarettes and the like; those ate the dos and the don'ts).

Chapter

THE NEARNESS OF BIRTH

After the frequent exams, the small fetus resembled a human being. It was becoming evident to both of us that the baby was on its way.

These were the things that began to happen to me at this moment:

A HEIGHTENED SENSE OF WHAT WAS TO COME

Things started to become more concrete to me around the fifth month of the pregnancy. Hearing the baby's heartbeat, even if it didn't sound like a genuine heart, was by far the most reassuring. Having the doctor try to convince me that what I was hearing was, in fact, a heartbeat, and a healthy one, made me feel a lot better.

THEN CAME THE DULLNESS

At this time, I was surrounded by ambiguity. I wasn't overjoyed about the pregnancy. And you don't have to judge yourself if you're in this situation. Some of us are terrified that something awful will happen to your partner or the baby, or that you will be caught in traffic when the delivery date approaches. Many unpleasant thoughts may arise.

Some people perceive the whole affair as an inconvenient waste of time and money. Others are concerned about losing their sex life, youth, freedom, friends, finances, and coveted position as the center of their partner's universe. Often, feelings of ambivalence or lack of interest are accompanied by guilt for not being more helpful or a better husband. Or a dread that these less-than-warm-and-fuzzy sensations are solid evidence that you'll be a bad father. All you need to do now is to take a rest.

Here are some of the things I tried to reduce the influence of ambivalence on me.

- Ask yourself, "Are you financially ready for parenthood (whatever that may mean to you), or are you merely concerned about money?"

- Are you completely prepared to be a father, or do you believe you were coerced into it? Have you completed everything you intended to accomplish at this point in your life, or are you resting on a pile of unfulfilled dreams?

- Is your spouse the lady of your dreams, or are you being pushed into your relationship? Similarly, is this the partnership of a lifetime, or do you have a hunch it won't last?

As you can probably guess, the more ambivalence you feel, the less you will feel invested during the rest of the pregnancy.

SOMETIMES YOU MIGHT FEEL LEFT OUT

While being more conscious of the reality of pregnancy is a positive thing, it is not the only thing that I felt around this time. Toward the conclusion of the third trimester, my wife began to focus more on what was going on inside her body, wondering if she'd be a good enough mother for this one, if he'd grow up to enjoy his mother more, and all the other tedious things that tend to irritate us fathers at this stage.

My wife was bonding with the baby at this moment. She was anxious about the baby's health or that every ache and agony she felt was a sign that the baby was in jeopardy. She was internalizing her sentiments about all of this as well, and at one point it appeared as if I didn't exist, which was rather disturbing. She was more focused on the baby inside her. Also, her mother paid her regular visits, and the two of them immediately formed a relationship with the baby.

So, if you find yourself in this circumstance, don't panic. Your wife isn't running away from you; what she's doing is normal. The concern is that while your spouse is turning inward, spending more time with her friends, or connecting with her own mother and the baby, you may wind up feeling left out, like I did when I didn't know better. But no matter how much it hurts, you must avoid the impulse to "retaliate" by withdrawing from her.

Make sure you're constantly soothing in a non-confrontational manner; don't let your emotions get the best of you in this circumstance; I know it hurts, but you'll need to understand and go with the flow. That is the biggest thing that has helped me in this scenario.

You can imagine how I felt when I watched various faces paying her a visit, while I was invisible to her. There were times when the only way she could remember me was to ask me to pass her the water bottle. I honestly considered asking her right there and then why she was treating me this way, why she made me feel nonexistent—but I'm glad I didn't, since I later discovered that they were among the factors that decreased her stress levels and allowed her to deliver a wonderful baby.

If you consider retaliating in any manner, you may trigger complications that might lead to miscarriage. And you know we don't want that. At this point, the baby will be so sensitive that anything the mother does on the outside will be felt by the baby. And, while it may seem strange to suggest a baby understands when it isn't wanted and may choose death or harming the mother within, which might result in a miscarriage, this is a consideration to keep in mind.

BE HER DOCTOR, BE HER SUPPORT

For some men, especially those who are feeling emotionally excluded by their partners, the excitement they feel at the developing reality of the pregnancy may be overwhelmed by their resentment at the way their partner's physicians treat them.

Some physicians can be irritating. Those sidelong looks that physicians give you when they're talking with your partner, making you feel like an invader, may be unpleasant, but the only thing we should concentrate on is taking care of our partner.

But did you know you have the power to not feel like a stranger at this point? Don't worry about how the doctor appears to you, as if they are trying to say, "*What are you doing here, please leave the room.*" Don't force it. Whether you know it or not, you probably have some clear ideas about how you want the pregnancy or birth to go—like I did, which lessened the strain I was feeling by ninety-nine percent.

So, what am I trying to express here? The simple reality is that if you are reduced to nothing more than a spectator, you will almost likely not receive what you desire. I recall well when this incident occurred to me, but it was when my wife's baby bump wasn't evident, and the doctor was giving her some advice on her vaginal health and the like.

"So, madam, you'll need to take care of yourself since there will be a lot of secretion at this time..." The doctor then peered at me with those corner eyes once again.

My wife looked at me. "Don't worry, doctor," she assured her. "He's my spouse, and I want him to stay."

The doctor continued. Well, you'll have a lot of secretions," she added, her expression solemn as she peered at me with her unpleasant corner eyes. "Make sure you clean the vagina thoroughly so that it doesn't produce an infection in the uterine canal." My wife was so absorbed that she didn't see how the doctor looked at me.

So, what am I trying to express here? If your wife wants you there, then stay there no matter what! Yes, a lot of males are a little squeamish about it, or feel uncomfortable when it comes to gynecological issues, and many hide in the corner to avoid having to deal with it. Remember, you are there for her. Set your feelings aside and be a man!

And, if your spouse has a male OB, it might be strange to be in the room as another guy puts his hands in regions you thought were off limits to everyone else. Pelvic examinations are normal medical procedures, and if you attend enough sessions, you will become accustomed to them. More and more, fathers are being embraced into the fold in recent years, but not nearly enough. In my situation, the OB doctor was acting like a jerk.

SYMPATHETIC PREGNANCY

"Wait a minute, isn't that for my wife?" you may think. That is reserved for you. This is a mental concern that many would-be dads confront throughout this stage of pregnancy.

"Oh my!" One morning, my wife woke me up. "You're packing on the pounds, sweetheart. "Are you stressed?" she said as she prepared herself a smoothie.

"Please," I begged. "You could have asked me to make you a smoothie, or one of our angels would have done it for you."

"I'm pregnant, sweetheart, not disabled," she remarked as she drank her smoothie while still staring at me. "All that weight, I suppose you quit working out?" she joked.

I checked myself out. "I'm not that big," I explained. At this time, my trousers were tearing up, so I knew she was telling the truth.

This is known as "Sympathetic syndrome," or, to use a scientific term, "Couvade." But I'm fine with "Sympathetic syndrome," because it emphasizes the argument I'm about to make.

The majority of what we men go through throughout the pregnant stage is psychological, which eventually leads to physical ailments. Various studies suggest that up to ninety percent of American expecting fathers experience this "Sympathetic syndrome," which is the same symptoms as pregnant women. Weight gain, mood swings, migraines, toothaches, and food cravings are all possible.

FEELING GUILTY

My wife raced out of the house one morning, clutching her tummy. It was ordinary morning sickness. I was standing behind her at the moment, and I couldn't bear how much she was going through because of me.

"Are you okay, my love?" I said, and then pulled up a seat for her, so she could sit and regain her breath. She was panting so hard this time that I was afraid.

"I need water," she remarked, so I handed her some. She grabbed the cup, drank the water, washed her mouth, and dumped it on the garden.

"Honey, let me lift..." I started, and she offered me a hand to halt.

She then turned to me, red. "I told you I didn't want this," she said, holding her stomach. "I told you to wear a condom, but you refused, stating you wanted to feel better."

"But..." I pleaded.

"Don't you act so sweet with me," she said. "You put me in this situation, and I feel like the baby is going to tear me apart."

"I'm very sorry, sweetie," I said. "Don't worry, once the baby arrives, none of this will matter.

"I know, but this one is a warrior," she whispered gently as she clutched her tummy. "That's what he's been doing, the tiny warrior has been hitting my walls."

I laughed. "Wait, he's going to be a hard slapper, right?" I was grinning from ear to ear.

My wife merely stared at me. "Do you think this is funny?" she inquired.

I kept my mouth shut. I knew I wasn't supposed to say anything that might aggravate her further. I absorbed all of the insults, but whenever I watched her in misery, I felt bad for making her this way.

Men have always been taught to bear pain and discomfort. And when our loved ones are in agony and we are unable to stop it, our natural, if a little misguided, reaction is to attempt to alleviate their suffering. To make it ours instead of theirs.

This is especially true if we have even the slightest sense, however irrational, that we are to blame for the pain in the first place. If your spouse has been experiencing morning sickness or other pregnancy-related difficulties, you may believe it is your responsibility. And, if her symptoms have been particularly severe, she may even encourage your subconscious guilt by telling you that you are the one who "got her into all of this" in the first place.

JEALOUSY

My mother and mother-in-law entered the house a few days later. I was glad to see both, but the moment I stepped forward, the first thing they asked for was my wife.

"Where is she?" my mother inquired. "The poor soul will be suffering from all those stomachaches."

"You know, right?" my wife's mother asked. "I remember she was all problems when I still had her in my stomach." They both laughed and continued to talk, completely unaware that I was present. That enraged me.

There is no doubt that your spouse will receive far more attention than you will during the pregnancy. And some men who acquire "sympathetic syndrome" symptoms do so Subconsciously to shift the attention of the pregnancy to themselves.

They were both in the room with my wife now, softly stroking her hands as she lay on the bed, feeling a lot more at ease with them there.

"Hello?" I motioned for attention. "Can't you see I'm right here?"

Both women turned to face me and waved me off. It was quite nasty, and I couldn't help but pant in envy. I observed how they handled my wife as if she was the only one who had a delicate heart, as if she was the only one who had been burdened by all the troubles in the previous months. Don't I have feelings? Is it expected that I wallow in it all? These ideas kept collapsing inside me. And I couldn't believe my mother was in on it.

"Hey, grab her some water, she's thirsty," my mother remarked.

"Mom!" I whined like a boy.

"You haven't outgrown this immature attitude of yours," my mother stated emphatically. "Get your wife some water to drink, or I'll pinch your ears if you still want to remain a child."

I marched into the kitchen, opened the fridge, and poured some water into a cup. I grew enraged, wondering why everyone was focusing on her. I knew it was right, but there was a part of me that couldn't help but be envious.

After a few minutes, I brought the water, and my wife drank to her heart's content. "I like the flavor of the water," she remarked. "Mom, why does the water taste… sweet?"

Seriously! She was now addressing my mother as her mother. The longer I saw this in front of me, the more irritated I became, and it got THIS CLOSE to me screaming at the top of my lungs for the attention I needed from these three women.

"What did you prepare for her?" her mother asked. "You know how important it is for the newborn to eat well?"

I'm not a nanny, I'm her husband, for Christ's sake, and I deserved the same care that they were providing her. They continued petting her, making me groan with jealousy. I finally decided to redirect, and finish reading my CIA spy book that I had started a few days prior.

So, what is my suggestion here? All you must do is completely adjust your focus. Start events that are appropriate for your current situation. You may start a project or accomplish something meaningful.

Lessons

- Mood swings and all are natural during this time. So why punish yourself?

- Don't guilt-trip yourself, guy; it's not worth it.

Chapter

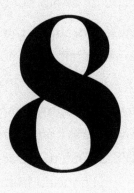

8

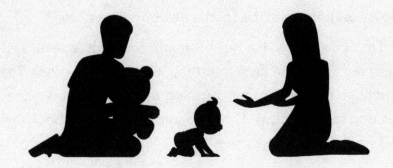

THE ARRIVAL: THE BIRTH OF OUR SON

My wife was in horrible pain in the afternoon, and the baby was already due. Fortunately, we had planned for it a few days beforehand. We were at the hospital when the staff started scurrying around looking for paperwork, injections, and medicines for my wife's birth.

"Ahhhhhhh," she yelled at the top of her lungs as she was transported by a stretcher. "It hurts so much!"

"Baby, take it easy, we'll be out of here soon," I reassured her as she was taken to the chamber we'd created.

"I don't think I can do this," she said right away. "The baby is kicking me so hard."

"Take a deep breath," I told her as she gripped the covers beneath her. She attempted to inhale with me for a few minutes before screaming again.

"It's not working!" she yelled. "Remove him from me!" she implored the nurses.

"We would do that, madam," the nurse answered, clearly nervous. "Take command; you will need to command the circumstance."

"How am I going to have control in this situation?" She shouted again. "The baby isn't giving me a chance." Then she took a deep breath in. "Please, baby boy, don't kick your mother like that..." And he kicked again, as if our little boy was taking no chances because he wanted to be free.

The entire labor process on average lasts around twelve to twenty hours—on the high end for first babies and on the low end for successive births—but there are no hard and fast rules. Labor is often separated into three phases. As I've discovered, the initial step also contains three stages.

STAGE 1

Phase 1 [Early or Latent labor]:

This is the longest portion of the labor, which can last anywhere from a few hours to a few days (but on average it is about eight hours). Fortunately, you'll be at home for most of it. Your spouse may not be able to feel the contractions, or the baby move at first. Even if she can, she'll probably tell you that they're manageable. These contractions typically last thirty to sixty seconds and can occur up to twenty minutes apart. They'll progressively become longer (sixty to ninety seconds), stronger, and closer together during the next several hours (perhaps as little as five minutes apart).

Every woman will have a somewhat different early labor experience. My wife experienced twelve hours of very lengthy contractions virtually every day for a week before our baby was born. Your spouse may also have "bloody show," which includes blood-tinged vaginal discharge, diarrhea, and backaches.

Phase 2 [Active Labor]:

This phase is often shorter (three to five hours), but significantly more intense than the first. If you're having a male, it might last up to ten minutes or longer than if you're having a girl. If you haven't already, go to the hospital. During the early stages of this period, your spouse will be able to chat through the contractions. They'll become closer (two or three minutes apart), longer, and stronger. She will begin to experience considerable agony as this stage advances. The bloody show will intensify and turn redder, and your partner will become less conversational as she focuses on the baby moving or the contractions.

"Honey, my stomach hurts," my wife said. "These contractions haven't stopped for three hours." Then she'd frown and look at me.

"All right," I murmured, my gaze fixed on her.

"Ouch," she said. "I feel the baby prodding me."

"Okay, let's get dressed," I said. "You don't have to wear this."

"I don't want to get dressed," she stated gently. "This is not the time to get dressed up."

"Come on, hon," I whimpered. "You don't have to be pissed."

"I'm not furious," she remarked as she touched her stomach softly. "I'm only expressing the obvious. You appear to be making the dumbest of decisions at this moment. "What do my contractions have to do with getting dressed?"

"You're wearing a nightgown. "How about putting some shoes and socks on?" I kept going.

"I don't want that," she stated once again. "You're irritating me!"

"But it's chilly out there," I said again. "How about a jacket?" I continued. Please do not decline the jacket."

"I don't want a jacket," she refused again.

"What in the world do you want?" I whimpered as I rose up in protest.

"What I need now is a cup of juice," she stated as she continued to touch her tummy.

Phase 3 [Transition]:

This normally lasts one or two hours. And once it starts, you'll understand why it's called "labor."

The baby moving in your partner may be practically unstoppable, lasting up to ninety seconds. And with just two or three minutes between the start of one and the start of the next contraction, there is hardly any time to recuperate in between. The agony is excruciating, and if your spouse is going to request medicines, this is most likely when she will do so. She's fatigued, sweating, her muscles are hurting and shaking, and she may be vomiting.

STAGE 2 [PUSHING AND BIRTH]

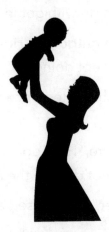

"Madam, you will have to push!" pleaded the doctor.

My wife wailed. "I can't," she said as she shook her head. "It's really uncomfortable."

"No, don't say that; if you claim your mind is painful, we won't leave this location," the doctor said. "Please be powerful and take command."

"MMMMMMMMMMMMM," she sang as she struggled to push.

"We're almost there, I can see a head," the doctor said. "Come on, keep pushing that baby out."

She hummed loudly again and attempted to push, then paused to rest.

Stage 2 is by far the most intense portion of the process—and thankfully for your partner it only lasts around two hours. Your partner's contractions or the baby moving within her are still long, lasting more than sixty seconds, but they are farther apart. The difference is that during the contractions, she will feel compelled to push, which is akin to wanting to urinate. She may feel some painful pressure and stinging when the baby's head "crowns" or kicks and begins to emerge through the vagina. But when the baby eventually comes out, there will be a big sense of relief.

Stage 3 [After the birth]

"It's out!" The doctor extracted my son, slithering out. The doctor then handed our son to the nurse. The nurses hurried for wipes and other supplies to clean the infant. But my wife didn't stop spilling everything out of her. The doctor removed the placenta and all other fluids let out as my wife was silently asleep.

"That's good," the doctor replied, and the nurse gave the infant a little slap on the buttocks, causing him to whimper.

We were all relieved when we heard that cry. The baby had come.

MY SITUATION

Starting labor was not easy for either my wife or me. As a result, she began to experience some bodily discomfort.

And, when she was screaming her heart out in that labor room, I was experiencing some psychological distress.

As soon as we were finished with the procedure, the doctor came, and the baby was cleaned up. And everything else I'd seen in that room that was a mess.

"Can I see her now?" I spoke up.

"You can, she's resting with the baby, "the doctor remarked.

The most essential thing to remember about this last stage of pregnancy is that the pain will fade. Her healing, though, will take an average of 6-8 weeks after birth. Possibly shorter, or longer.

BABY, BABY

It was time for my fatherly duties. My child was a bundle of delight to me, and finally holding my son made me... soft on the inside. I felt successful, and I couldn't help but smile from ear to ear as I looked at this bundle of pleasure before me.

The infant then started crying. Those feelings of psychological guilt reared its ugly head again the moment he began to cry.

Babies have six distinct behavioral states that are visible within a few minutes of birth. So, by recognizing them and comprehending when they occur and what anticipated reactions are in each, parents can not only learn to know their newborns but also give the most responsiveness for their requirements.

In my first few weeks as a new father, I discovered that understanding these states was a big assistance in getting to know my baby. Here's a rundown of the six states and how I acted in each.

ACTIVE ALERT

The baby is in its cot and begins to make little sounds and move his arms, head, torso, and face, as well as his eyes, regularly and aggressively.

"WRRRR," the infant will exclaim. "Gaggagaaa."

The baby's movements are generally brief—a few seconds of activity per minute or two. According to some studies, these motions are intended to provide parents with subtle cues about what their child wants and needs. Others argue that these motions are just entertaining to observe and hence encourage parent-infant contact.

QUIET ALERT

When I checked on the baby this time, it was all motionless, wide-eyed, and staring at me. When it heard a footstep or something drop, it would shiver, pick up the sensory inputs, and remain alert.

Babies in a calm alert state do not move much since all of their energy is concentrated on seeing and listening. They are unable to follow items with their eyes and will replicate your facial expressions.

Most babies have a forty-minute phase of quiet alertness or silent alertness within their first hour of life. During his or her first week, the average newborn spends approximately ten percent of any twenty-four-hour period in this condition. This is by far the coolest state, the period when your child is most interested in and absorbing knowledge about his or her new surroundings. This is also the period when you and your child will have your first few moments of connection, when you will realize that there is a real person within that little body.

CRYING

I remember carrying the baby and wanting to give him some milk his mother had pumped into a bottle. The guy screamed and cried, and I was frantic because I didn't know what was going on.

"Oh, give me that," his mother said, still lying on the bed.

"I think he doesn't like me," I said to my wife.

"No, don't say that sweetheart..."

And that is correct; I should not have reached that conclusion. Crying is quite normal, and for some, all too frequent. The infant's eyes may be open or closed, his face crimson, and his arms and legs writhing around.

Often, simply picking up the baby and walking about with him or her can cease the sobbing. And that's exactly what my wife did here.

"All you have to do is carry him around," she explained.

I was skeptical, but I decided to give it a shot. There was nothing to lose. So, I gently removed the infant from her arms and performed as she requested. It was a complete marvel that the infant went as quiet as a moth and just goggled words while staring at me with those deep blue eyes of his.

Surprisingly, psychologists used to believe that newborns were comforted because they loved being held upright. What truly makes them stop sobbing is movement or frequent rocking motions.

As uncomfortable as it might be at times, crying is not necessarily a bad thing; it not only helps the baby to communicate but also provides essential exercise. So, if your efforts to soothe him or her aren't immediately effective, and the baby isn't hungry or stewing in a filthy diaper, don't panic. The cries may stop on their own after a few minutes.

QUIET SLEEP

Another day, I came up to check on my son in his cot. But all I noticed was that he was still. When I called my wife, she hobbled into the room.

"What in the world is it?" she exclaimed, clutching her chest in terror.

"Isn't the baby supposed to move?" I inquired.

My wife looked at me, clearly annoyed.

"Please don't frighten me like that again, and leave the young guy to sleep," she limped out of the room. "He's okay."

The baby's face was perfectly calm, and his eyes were still

closed and in the "Quiet Sleep" state. His body would scarcely move at all, though his mouth quivered nearly imperceptible from time to time.

Babies in the quiet sleep stage sleep very peacefully—so soundly asleep that the absence of movement and inaudible breathing can startle you. If this occurs, all you need to do is lean in close and listen for the baby's breath. Otherwise, place a gentle palm on his chest—you should always lay your baby to sleep on his back and watch his breathing rise and fall. Try to avoid the desire to poke the baby to see whether she's still alive—most babies spend up to ninety percent of their first few weeks asleep.

LIGHT SLEEP (REM SLEEP)

This time I arrived to feed him. I called his name softly, but he was fast asleep, grunting and smiling.

"Oh, little buddy, do you have dreams?" I was taken aback and could only watch him for an hour as he played in his own dream.

The baby's eyes are normally closed, but he may grin or frown, make sucking or chewing movements, and even moan or twitch, exactly like you do in your "active sleep" condition. If you look closely, you can see the eyeballs moving around behind the eyelids.

Sixty percent of a baby's sleep time is spent in silent sleep and forty percent in active sleep, with the two stages alternating back and forth. So, if your sleeping baby begins to stir, whimper, or appears to be waking up unhappy, wait a few seconds before picking him up to feed, change, or comfort. If left alone, the infant may go back into a deep slumber.

For thousands of years, most people thought that newborns could simply feed, sleep, wail, and gaze about. However, if you pay attention, you will see that your new baby has an extraordinary arsenal of abilities.

Your baby is already communicating with you and everyone else around him after only a few hours out of the womb. He can replicate your facial expressions, has some control over his body, can express preferences—the most liked are patterned items over plain objects and curved lines over straight ones—and has a phenomenal memory.

However, if you want your baby to interact and play with you, the time to do it is during the active alert stage. Babies are especially sensitive to strong contrast during the first few months, hence black and white toys and patterns are frequently popular. But you must be patient. Babies are highly intelligent, but they also have their own minds. This implies that, despite your best efforts, your baby may not be interested in performing with you—yes, a baby can perform with you; in this stage, if you stick your tongue out, they'll copy what you're doing. Babies are very intellectual beings.

WHAT HAPPENED WITH US AFTERWARD

My wife and I began to bond more after our son was born. I felt a sense of peace return to me, and I was relieved that all the trouble of going here and there looking for info and answers had passed. And it appeared that my wife had forgotten all that she had happened in the previous several months; all she was concerned with was being a mother and providing more for her newest child.

I didn't want to go back to work at that time. And I knew how to make that happen. All I had to do to spend a couple extra months with my family was ask my supervisor for some leave. My boss and I had a good relationship, so he knew I was prompt and dedicated to my job.

On a certain day, I phoned in sick.

"Hello, boss," I said as I strolled into his office. He smiled the moment he saw me.

"And here comes the new father," he remarked. "How are you?"

My heart was racing, and I could feel the adrenaline rush. "I'm okay, sir," I explained.

He came over to give me a light hug—yes, he was that close to me.

"Please, please, have a seat," he urged, taking his own seat. "So, what brings you to the office? I thought you were utilizing this time to bond with the baby a little."

"Yes, sir," I answered, my hands wet and softly stroking them over my jeans while sitting. "I came here expressly for it."

He paid attention. "Don't tell me you want to quit your job?" he demanded. I could see he was tense.

"No, that's not it," I responded, and he exhaled in relief. I knew it would be a loss to the establishment if I left; I was one of the most loyal employees, and I had worked tirelessly to keep this business operating.

"So, what do you want?" he said. "Tell me anything, and I'll do it."

I grinned, feeling a little more at ease now. "I'll need to request a leave, sir," I explained. "I want to use this opportunity to reconnect with my family."

He gave me a brief smile before turning to face me. "Is that why you were so silent when you came in?"

I nodded.

"Well, you have the rest of the month to yourself." He added, "I'll also throw in some goodies to help you get through this."

My heart leaped and I gasped. "Really, sir?" I murmured, my eyes wide with delight, and he nodded.

I offered my hand for a shake, and he firmly grasped it. "Thank you very much, sir," I said.

"No, we need to thank you for being here when we needed you the most," he explained.

"I am very grateful," I said.

"Don't worry," he said. "When you go, I'll inform the bank to initiate the proceedings."

I left the workplace feeling light. My coworkers were all congratulating me and offering to pay me a visit to see the baby.

PATERNAL FEELING

Despite the excitement, you may feel a sense of peace and harmony. You might not want to go to work and would rather spend time with your new family. If so, you are not alone.

Anne Storey, a researcher, discovered that new fathers' testosterone levels frequently decline by a third shortly after the birth of their children. Storey speculates that this type of testosterone drop might make a guy feel more paternal or like "settling down."

Lessons

- A newborn is a delight, so pay attention to how they behave, and act accordingly.

Chapter

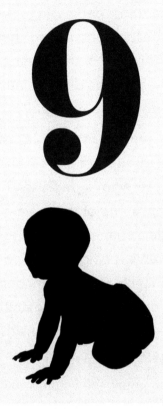

9

THE FATHER FEELING AND ALL THINGS BABY

POSTPARTUM DEPRESSION

Yes, I felt depressed around a month after the child was delivered. I recall having a searing headache after calculating the expense of the baby's food, diapers, and other necessities. Then my wife walked into the room to ask me a question. I snapped, and immediately started yelling and said "I'm in the middle of calculating our finances, can you come back later!

What I want to tell you now is that this can happen sometimes. Postpartum depression symptoms include emotions of stress, despair, and anger. There is an aversion to hearing the baby cry, hatred of the infant and all the attention he or she receives, as well as disappointment and tiredness about how you are doing as a new dad.

While no one understands what causes postpartum depression, certain groups of males are more vulnerable than others. A spouse who is depressed or has a personal history of depression is one of the most obvious risk factors. Other factors include a financial crisis, a poor connection with your spouse or parents, being unmarried, or an unplanned or undesired pregnancy. Postpartum depression does not discriminate based on socioeconomic status or race. It usually affects first-time parents, although it can arise with subsequent deliveries even if there were no symptoms with the first.

If you feel you may be suffering from postpartum depression, know that it is not a show of weakness. It does not make you a terrible father or imply that you do not love your child. It is a recognized medical issue that affects hundreds of thousands of fathers, and you should not have to suffer when therapy is available.

Much more commonly is Post Partem Depression in the mother. This is a very real possibility for new mothers, and it should be taken seriously. Be sure to keep your heart open for your partner if she shows signs of post partem depression and help her find a support system to help her through this.

BONDING WITH THE BABY

Nobody knows when it began, but one of the most common and lasting fallacies about child rearing is that women are more caring than males and hence better suited to parenting.

That is not true since men are just as concerned, engaged, and invested in their infants as mothers are. We also hold, touch, kiss, rock, and coo at our new kids with at least the same frequency as mothers do.

"Honey, you're making me jealous," my wife said to me one day as she watched me play with the baby.

"Why," I said, laughing heartily.

"You're all on the baby, and you're even neglecting me here," she said.

"No, sweetie," I answered. "You are my world, but the baby takes priority."

My wife gasped and punched me playfully, and we started laughing at each other. It was such a happy time. And if it were possible to wish, I would wish for that moment again and again, even though we've shared so many other beautiful moments.

UNFEELING PARENTS

This doesn't sit well with me, but I've heard that it does happen. Where either the mother or father does not feel a connection to their newborn. Some even put them away and refuse to feed the baby, causing it to cry until it is sick.

Few people will openly admit in public that they have no feelings for their infant. Doesn't it sound creepy? But it does exist.

Indeed, according to academics Kay Robson and Ramesh Kumar, forty percent of moms and dads who participated in their study reported they had no feelings for their child. Only complete disinterest.

There are a variety of reasons for this, including the parents' belief that they do not know the baby well enough or that the infant does not look like them or the agony the spouse felt during labor or delivery was caused by the baby, among other things.

With all these factors, all I can say is don't blame yourself if you discover you have no feelings for the infant. No, don't push it too far or feel as if you've been mistreated as a parent or mother. All you need to do is take your time, don't put too much pressure on yourself, and don't consider for a second that you've failed as a parent. Almost all new fathers experience that connecting sense within two months.

There is a lot of evidence that physical intimacy fosters parent-child connection. So, if you want to speed up the process, consider carrying the baby whenever possible, taking him with you whenever possible, and taking care of as many of his basic requirements as feasible.

If you have twins, bonding will most likely be more difficult. Multiples may need to stay in the hospital nursery for a few days or even weeks because they are delivered prematurely, limiting the amount of time you can spend with them–separately or together. Things can get even more problematic if one of the babies comes home with you while the other(s) stays behind. You'll be pulled between spending time with the baby in the hospital, the other baby, and your partner. Unfortunately, there is no secret formula for determining how much time each of them receives. All you can do is try your best to spend time chatting with your spouse about how you're feeling and what each of you need.

HOW TO STAY INVOLVED

"Honey," my wife complained.

"Yes, baby," I replied as I rocked my newborn in my arms.

"You're so focused on the baby, and you've failed to listen to my needs," she acted like a kid.

"Is my poodle-hon angry?" I said my normal lovely phrases.

And she produced a silly frown. "You know it's our baby, but you can still pretend you love me more," she explained.

And I laughed. "Well, I'm simply gazing at the man who is going to transform the world for the better," I said to my youngster. "I'm going to teach him sports, science, cooking, and a lot of other things my father taught me as a kid."

My wife grinned. "I'd be overjoyed if our son turns out like his father," she remarked. "It would be the finest blessing." At this time, we both glanced at each other and gave each other a light peck on the lips.

You'll have to learn to manage many roles in the first few days. You're still a lover and friend to your spouse, and of course you're a parent, but for the time being, your most essential position is that of a support person to your partner. Aside from her physical recuperation, she'll need some time to get to know the baby and learn (if she wishes) how to nurse.

Lessons

- Postpartum Depression exists, and you should be aware of it.

- Connect with your baby, connect, connect, connect.

Chapter

10

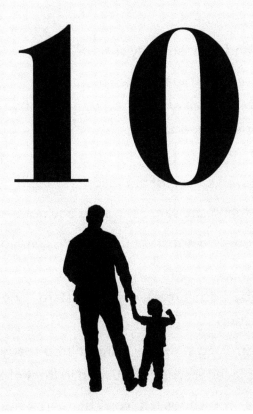

FATHERHOOD

I was the support person for my spouse for the first several weeks and months after the birth of my child, and you will experience the same thing.

"Have you eaten, honey?" I inquired as I was preparing something in the kitchen.

"No, sweetheart," she answered, swiping through her phone. "The majority of my Facebook friends are wishing me luck. "I'm on top of the world right now."

I burst out laughing.

"Really, and what are they saying?" I asked.

"Well, "I am very pleased for you, lady," by MaryAnn Kumbo from Kenya, "the baby is a cutie," by Toby Igbo from Nigeria," she proceeded to read.

"Well, that's quite beautiful," I observed as I entered the living room with a bowl of her favorite custard.

"What's that?" she said as soon as she noticed the custard.

"Come on, sweetheart," I urged. "It'll give you the energy you need."

"But, baby, I don't really need a custard," she explained. "I need lamb soup."

"We're creating it for you, and it'll be ready in a flash," I added as I placed a scoop of custard in front of her.

Whatever you choose, it won't be long before you realize that being a parent in America, especially an involved one, is not an easy job. This is why I always tip my hat to my father; he was a superman. I'm not sure how he did it, but he managed to sustain the family for a long period. The task of the work is arduous and at times irritating, but the largest challenges you'll encounter are the ones they neglected to tell you previously, namely the societal ones.

And it is only in the last few decades that men and women have been free to speak out against the conventional position of dads in the family. And it is only recently that society has understood that remote dads are seldom perfect fathers. But, in the middle of this newfound freedom to strike out against yesterday's absent, negligent dads, today's fathers—that's you—are falling victim to old prejudices.

According to misconceptions, men have not taken an active role in family life because they don't want to. But is this still true today? Hardly. More and more of us are realizing that traditional metrics of success aren't all they're made up to be, and we're dedicated to being a physical and emotional presence in our children's lives. In one study, most men between the ages of twenty and forty-five believe that having a work schedule that allows them to spend more time with their families is more essential than undertaking tough job or even earning a high wage. And many of these guys would willingly forget money in exchange for more family time. The issue is that society not only does not support us but actively discourages us.

Frankly put, Americans are not as interested in fatherhood as they are in motherhood—even the terms conjure up distinct images: motherhood is caring, nurturing, and loving, whereas fatherhood is simply a biological bond. As a result, males are rarely accepted if they play a different role than the one, they are "supposed" to play.

The focus on a typical job begins early. Even before they can walk, children of both sexes are inundated with the notion that dads are essentially unnecessary.

Without further ado, let me share some of the strategies I devised and used to engage my children:

- *Start it Dude:*

If you don't start taking the lead, there's no way in hell you'll ever be able to accept the child-bearing obligations you desire, and your children deserve. Instead of allowing your partner to remove a wailing or stinky baby from your arms, consider saying something like, "No, honey, let me handle this," or "Wait a minute, this is easy." There's also nothing wrong with seeking guidance if you need it. You each have insights that the other may use. However, instead of doing it for you, have her inform you.

- *Get some support:*

Even before your baby is born, you're likely to become aware of the numerous support groups for new moms. It won't take you long to discover, however, that there are few, if any, organizations for new dads. And if you do find one, it will most likely be aimed at guys whose interaction with their children is restricted to five minutes before sleep.

- *If you're in a position to do something for other folks, do it:*

All else being equal, try hiring a male babysitter occasionally, or consider asking a guy friend to babysit instead of the typical female pals when you or your wife desire a night away. If you need to ease into it, consider the responsible teenage son of some friends. Continuing to distrust men and boys will keep them thinking of themselves as untrustworthy, making it difficult for them to feel comfortable enough in their role as parents to take on as much responsibility as they—and their partners—would want.

- **Keep the communication:**

If you don't like the current situation, you can tell your partner, but please be nice. Do not take it personally if she initially appears hesitant to share the job of parent with you. Men aren't the only ones who have struggled with socialization. Many women have been conditioned to think that if they are not the primary caregivers—even if they work outside the home—they have failed as moms.

So, in this situation, in my view, and I hope your spouse is reading this as well, until men are recognized as parents, the responsibility of childbearing will fall disproportionately on women, frustrating their efforts to achieve equality.

- **Get Involved in your kids' day-to-day lives:**

This simply means making an extra effort to share tasks like meal planning, grocery shopping, cooking, taking the kids to the library or bookstore, getting to know their classmates and parents, and organizing playdates with your spouse. Not doing these things might create the appearance that you don't believe they're essential or that you're not interested in being an involved parent. And by doing so, you increase the likelihood that your spouse will feel comfortable and secure in sharing the nurturing role with you. But make an effort to spend some "quality" time alone with the kids as well. Sure, someone needs to drive the kids across town to medical visits, taekwondo courses, piano lessons, ballet lessons, or soccer practice, but that shouldn't be your sole interaction with them.

HERE'S WHERE I DROP THE PEN

Throughout this book, we've discussed my own experiences and the benefits—both to you and your children—of being an active, involved father, as well as how fatherhood begins well before your first child is born. The one thing we haven't discussed is the beneficial impact your parenting role may have on your relationship with your partner.

So, this book is all about experiencing and loving every stage of parenthood, especially when the baby is born. The happiness you feel and what you are bound to feel as time passes. The cost and all the essentials might be a pain in the neck for us fathers at times, but once the child is born and developing right before your eyes, you fill up with progress.

Also remember that those who provide help must also look after themselves. Giving and giving to your lover can be exhausting and emotionally draining. So, while you go through this pregnancy and birth with your spouse, remember to practice self-care.

Pregnancy or motherhood is a time for your spouse to take care of her emotional needs, consume nutritious meals, exercise, and avoid bad behaviors like drinking and smoking. This might be a chance for you to do the same, giving you the stamina to be the strong, emotional partner you require right now.

Most importantly, if you are feeling overwhelmed, nervous, or sad, you should know that you are not alone, and that assistance is available if you require it. Share your emotions with your spouse, friends, and family. You may also want to talk to a counselor, therapist, or your healthcare practitioner about taking further actions to improve your mental and emotional health.

What makes you think you can't do it the same way I did it? Pregnancy and childbirth may be the most beautiful experiences, but only if you set your mind to it and don't let doubt or despair creep in and make you think adversely about the situation.

In addition, and perhaps most importantly, you will need to be the ideal father to your children. *Be the parent they'll be happy to show off to their friends.*

And, yeah, you don't expect me to know all there is to know about gynecologists and obstetricians and all the jargon—I'll preserve my sources so you can look them up yourself; the references are below!

REFERENCES

Goetzl, L.M. "Clinical Management Guidelines for Obstetrician-Gynecologists Number, 36, July 2002. Obstetric analgesia and anesthesia." *Obstetrics & Gynecology 100. No. 1*

Hanson, Suzanne, Lauren, P. Hunter, et, al. "Paternal Fears of childbirth. A literature review." *Journal of Perinatal Education.*

Printed in the USA
CPSIA information can be obtained
at www.ICGtesting.com
LVHW012156020924
789950LV00033B/1478